Interferon
Properties, Mode of Action, Production, Clinical Application

Beiträge zur Onkologie
Contributions to Oncology

Vol. 11

Series Editors
S. Eckhardt, Budapest; *J. H. Holzner,* Wien;
G. A. Nagel, Göttingen

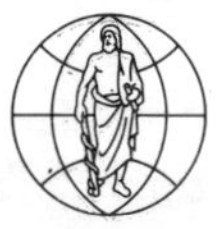

S. Karger · Basel · München · Paris · London · New York · Sydney

Proceedings of the 3rd International Expert Meeting of the Deutsche Stiftung für Krebsforschung, Bonn, March 13–16, 1981

Interferon

Properties, Mode of Action, Production, Clinical Application

Volume Editors
K. Munk and *H. Kirchner*, Heidelberg

50 figures and 70 tables, 1982

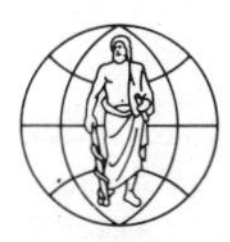

S. Karger · Basel · München · Paris · London · New York · Sydney

Beiträge zur Onkologie
Contributions to Oncology

Vol. 9: Adriamycin-Symposium. Ergebnisse und Aspekte. Gemeinsames Symposium der Arbeitsgemeinschaft Internistische Onkologie (AIO) der Deutschen Krebsgesellschaft und der Farmitalia Carlo Erba (Freiburg i. Br.), Frankfurt a. M. 1981
Herausgeber: D. Füllenbach, Freiburg i. Br.; G. A. Nagel, Göttingen; S. Seeber, Essen
X + 462 S., 110 Abb., 5 Farbt., 167 Tab., 1981. ISBN 3-8055-2966-X

Vol. 10: Plasmapheresis in Immunology and Oncology. Symposium of Arbeitsgemeinschaft Internistische Onkologie der Deutschen Krebsgesellschaft, Göttingen 1980
Editors: J. H. Beyer, Göttingen; H. Borberg, Köln; Ch. Fuchs, G. A. Nagel, Göttingen
VIII + 274 p., 86 fig., 44 tab., 1982. ISBN 3-8055-3467-1

National Library of Medicine, Cataloging in Publication
Interferon-properties, mode of action, production, clinical application: proceedings of a symposium, Bonn, March 13–16, 1981/volume editors, K. Munk and H. Kirchner. – Basel; New York: Karger, 1982
(Beiträge zur Onkologie; Bd. 11)
1. Interferon-congress I. Kirchner, H. II. Munk, K. III. Series
ISBN 3-8055-3482-5
WI BE444N Bd. 11
[QV 268.5 161 1981]

Drug Dosage

The author and publisher have exerted every effort to ensure that drug selection and dosage set forth in this text are in accord with current recommendations and practice at the time of publication. However, in view of ongoing research, changes in government regulations, and the constant flow of information relating to drug therapy and drug reactions, the reader is urged to check the package insert for each drug for any change in indications and dosage and for added warnings and precautions. This is particularly important when the recommended agent is a new and/or infrequently employed drug.

Printed in Germany
ISBN 3-8055-3482-5

Contents

Preface VII

Friedman, R. M.; Czarniecki, C. W.; Epstein, D. A. (Bethesda, Maryland); *Jay, F. T.* (Winnipeg, Manitoba); *Maheshwari, R. K.; Sreevalsan, T.* (Washington, D. C.), and *Panet, A.* (Jerusalem): Mechanisms of Interferon Action on Cell Growth and on Murine Leukemia, Vesicular Stomatitis, and Encephalomyocarditis Viruses 1

Jungwirth, C.; Strube, W.; Strube, M.; Kroath, H. (Würzburg), and *Graf, T.* (Heidelberg): Interferon Inhibits the Establishment of Fibroblast Infection by Avian Retroviruses 11

Lucero, M. A.; Magdelenat, H.; Fridman, W. H.; Pouillart, P.; Billardon, C. (Paris); *Billiau, A.* (Leuven); *Cantell, K.* (Helsinki), and *Falcoff, E.* (Paris): Pharmacological Properties of Human Alpha and Beta Interferons 17

Masucci, M. G.; Klein, E.; Masucci, G.; Szigeti, R., and *Vanky, F.* (Stockholm): Effect of Interferon on Certain Cellular Immune Functions 30

Borden, E. C.; Yamamoto, N.; Hogan, T. F.; Edwards, B. S., and *Bryan, G. T.* (Madison, Wisconsin): Interferons: Preclinical Rationale for Trials in Human Bladder Carcinoma 42

Fleischmann, W. R., Jr. (Galveston, Texas): Interferon Potentiation: Antiviral and Antitumor Studies 53

Pape, G. R.; Hadam, M. R.; Eisenburg, J., and *Riethmüller, G.* (München): Natural-Killer Cell Activation in Patients Following Human Interferon-Beta Therapy 63

De Maeyer-Guignard, J.; Dandoy, F., and *De Maeyer, E.* (Orsay): Host Genotype Influences Interferon Action in the Mouse 73

Burke, D. C. (Coventry, Warwickshire): A Monoclonal Antibody against Interferon-Alpha 83

Hochkeppel, H. K.; Menge, U., and *Collins, J.* (Braunschweig): Monoclonal Antibodies against Human Fibroblast Interferon 94

Sulkowski, E. (Buffalo, New York) and *Goeddel, D. V.* (South San Francisco, California): Hydrophobicity of Human Interferons 106

Berg, K.; Hokland, M., and *Heron, I.* (Aarhus): Biological Activities of Pure HuIFN-α Species 118

Knight, E., Jr.; Blomstrom, D. C. (Wilmington, Delaware), and *Hunkapiller, M. W.* (Pasadena, California): Characterization of Human (β) Fibroblast Interferon 127

Finter, N. B.; Allen, G.; Ball, G. D.; Fantes, K. H.; Johnston, M., and *Priestman, T.* (Beckenham, Kent): Studies with Lymphoblastoid Interferon 131

Wussow, P. von; Chen, M.; Platsoucas, C. D.; Wiranowska–Stewart, M., and *Stewart*, (New York): Production of Human Gamma Interferon for Clinical Trials 135

Krammer, P. H.; Kees, U.; Marcucci, F., and *Kirchner, H.* (Heidelberg): Immune Interferon Production by T-Cell Clones 144

Vilček, J.; Yip, Y. K. (New York), and *Pang, R. H. L.* (Rockville, Maryland): Induction and Characterization of Human Immune (Gamma) Interferon 150

Oettgen, H. F. and *Krown, S. E.* (New York): Clinical Trials of Human Leukocyte Interferon at the Memorial Sloan-Kettering Cancer Center 159

De Somer, P. (Leuven): Perspectives for Clinical Use of Fibroblast Interferon 173

Neumann-Haefelin, D.; Sundmacher, R. (Freiburg), and *Cantell, K.* (Helsinki): Corneal Interferon Treatment of Herpetic Keratitis in Monkeys 185

Sundmacher, R.; Neumann-Haefelin, D. (Freiburg), and *Cantell, K.* (Helsinki): The Clinical Value of Interferon in Ocular Viral Diseases 191

Müller, R. (Hannover); *Deinhardt, F.; Frösner, G.* (München); *Hofschneider, H. P.* (Martinsried); *Klein, H.; Schmidt, F. W.* (Hannover); *Siegert, W.* (München); *Wille, E.*, and *Vido, I.* (Hannover): Human Interferon-Beta in Chronic Active Hepatitis B: Preliminary Data of a Controlled Trial 197

Niethammer, D. and *Treuner, J.* (Tübingen): Experience with Fibroblast-Derived Interferon as an Antitumor Agent 205

Lampert, F.; Berthold, F. (Giessen); *Treuner, J.*, and *Niethammer, D.* (Tübingen): Therapeutical Trial for Neuroblastoma Stage IV (GPO-Study NBL-79) 213

Huhn, D.; Fink, U.; Theml, H.; Siegert, W.; Riethmüller, G., and Wilmanns, W. (München): Interferon in Non-Hodgkin-Lymphoma of Low Malignancy 217

Herfarth, Ch.; Schlag, P., and *Schreml, W.* (Ulm-Safranberg): Randomized Controlled Study to Examine the Effectiveness of Fibroblast Interferon as an Adjuvant Therapy in Gastric Carcinoma Operated for Cure 224

Strander, H. (Stockholm): Interferon Therapy for Tumor Diseases in Man: Prospects for the Near Future 227

Preface

The Deutsche Krebshilfe was founded by Dr. Mildred Scheel as a private foundation. The reaction and response of the German people to this foundation, which is dedicated to finding solutions for this urgent medical problem, has been very great. The Deutsche Krebshilfe received, throughout the years, money from individual private donors, legacies, and many other sources. The enthusiastic donations by the population have never ceased since the start of the foundation and continue in a way which gives reason to admire the goodwill of the people.

However, in regard to this money donated to the Deutsche Krebshilfe, there are, of course, great demands placed upon these persons, particularly on Dr. Scheel and her scientific and organizational advisors, and suggestions on how to make the best use of these donations. The people expect, of course, this money to be given to the discovery of solutions to the most urgent problems in the medical care of cancer and to the most fruitful projects in cancer research. In regard to this challenge, the Deutsche Krebshilfe always followed one main goal, that is the idea that a private foundation should always be innovative. It should always start and support projects which are new, which cannot be started because of the lack of official initiative, or because of the lack of official financial support, or because there are administrative barriers which inhibit or retard the tackling of urgent projects.

These goals, however, require the persistent efforts and the expertise of those who are asked to advise the Deutsche Krebshilfe. In addition, since the cancer problem is international and the fight against cancer needs a combined international effort, a comprehensive, world-wide group of experts is needed. The Deutsche Krebshilfe always sought the advice of international experts in order to help the foundation work best for the benefit of the cancer patients of today and tomorrow.

The meetings of experts, of which this was the third one, are examples for the international and comprehensive discussions on the aims and tasks of the Deutsche Krebshilfe. The idea to devote this meeting to interferon is Dr. Scheel's because she was frequently approached by patients to supply the financial means for individual interferon therapies. Since the interferon problem is, at present, extensively discussed within the community of scientists as well as the laypress, Dr. Scheel again sought the advice of internationally recognized experts in this field. She expects, from the results of this meeting, the best possible clarification and an expert evaluation of the significance of interferon therapy, particularly in comparison with other forms of cancer treatment. During the past year, the interferon field has exploded scientifically. Some of the dynamite workers involved were at this meeting.

The reasons for the enormous progress in interferon research have been basically threefold:

First, there have been breakthroughs in the protein chemistry and the molecular biology of interferon. Thus, it is now proven that interferons are a class of different proteins, and the amino acid sequence of some has been identified.

We want to stress the following: Interferons are a group of defined proteins with exceedingly high biologic activities in different systems.

Secondly, it has been possible to introduce and express the gene of human interferon in *E. coli*. This may be a promising way towards producing interferon in sufficient quantities. Most excitingly, the *E. coli* product seems to share many of the known properties of human interferon.

Thirdly, there has been a tremendous clinical interest in interferon due to the possibility that interferon may be of some use in the treatment of neoplastic disease.

Please note that we have used the term *may*. It was obviously one of the purposes of this meeting to achieve a critical evaluation of the available clinical data.

When a research field explodes, as it has happened to interferon research, people working in the field may have a twofold reaction, and this applies to those who have worked in the field for ten or more years, particularly our distinguished guests.

On the one side, it is a good feeling to realize that the scientific community finally acknowledges the importance of something of which we have been convinced for quite a while.

On the other side, one is afraid when there is too much uncritical enthusiasm, particularly when something as serious as the treatment of cancer is involved and when the lay-press begins to be interested.

Now, in this situation, we feel that we owe the public clear-cut statements about the state of affairs. Dr. Scheel is very concerned about these matters.

As it has happened often in cancer medicine, so-called new forms of therapy have raised much optimism, then failed, and subsequently seriously blocked future developments. In such situations, short-cuts to practical medicine have turned out to be disasters.

All of us are convinced that interferons are of tremendous biologic significance. Interferons may turn out to be of clinical value but we are far from having a sound evaluation on this point. We want to stress, however, that most likely no progress will be made unless the way is paved by thorough research in the laboratories. Clinical application of interferons would probably have never occurred if scientists did not treat mice with interferons about ten years ago. Similarly, we believe that future therapeutic improvements will depend on the progress made in laboratories. Furthermore, in regard to clinical studies, the *very least* we have to postulate is that therapeutical trials are accompanied by thorough clinical investigations so that we may learn more about the pharmacokinetics of interferons and many other things. Otherwise, the therapeutic trials may turn out to be useless and extremely costly.

The editors acknowledge the competent assistance of Ms. Marion Kasamasch.

Heidelberg, 1981

Klaus Munk
Holger Kirchner

Mechanisms of Interferon Action on Cell Growth and on Murine Leukemia, Vesicular Stomatitis, and Encephalomyocarditis Viruses

Robert M. Friedman[1], *Christine W. Czarniecki*[1], *David A. Epstein*[1], *Francis T. Jay*[1, 2], *Radha K. Maheshwari*[1, 3], *T. Sreevalsan*[4], *Amos Panet*[1, 5]

[1] National Institute of Arthritis, Metabolism, and Digestive Diseases, National Institutes of Health, Bethesda, Maryland, USA
[2] Department of Medical Microbiology, University of Manitoba, Winnipeg, Manitoba, Canada
[3] Interferon Laboratory, Howard University Cancer Center, Washington, D. C., USA
[4] Department of Microbiology, Georgetown University Medical & Dental Schools, Washington, D. C., USA
[5] Department of Virology, Hebrew University, Hadassah Medical School, Jerusalem, Israel

The basis for the antiviral activity of interferons in the case of a lytic virus like encephalomyocarditis virus (EMC) appears to be the inhibition of viral protein synthesis [1]. In contrast, the interferon-induced suppression of retroviruses, such as murine leukemia virus (MLV) in chronically infected cells, appears to occur at a late stage of virus growth [1]. In interferon-treated cells infected with mouse mammary tumor virus [2, 3] or MLV [4, 5, 6], virus yields are significantly inhibited. Inhibition of retrovirus production was not correlated with inhibition of at least some intracellular steps in virus replication [4, 5]. In interferon-treated AKR cells in which there was a marked decrease in the production of both endogenous MLV particles and infectious MLV, the intracellular concentration of viral p30 (group-specific) antigen was unaffected or even increased [5]. Synthesis of the viral proteins p30, gp69/71, and p15 was not inhibited in interferon-treated mouse 3T3 fibroblast cells infected with MLV; synthesis and cleavage of the precursors of these proteins were also unaffected [7]. In interferon-treated AKR cells, scanning electron and transmission micrographs, in fact, clearly indicated that in mouse systems the number of surface-associated MLV particles was increased [8, 9].

RNA synthesis by retroviruses has also been studied. In interferon-treated mouse cells infected with Moloney-MLV or AKR-MLV, the concentration of virus-specific RNA was approximately the same as in untreated cells. The rates of viral RNA synthesis were also about equal [6, 10]. Substantially the same findings have been made in chronic mouse mammary tumor virus infection after interferon treatment [3]. During inhibition by interferon of exogenous or endogenous infection, the findings were similar to those previously discussed in that the interferon block appeared to occur at or just before virus assembly so that, although there was no inhibition of viral p30 (group-specific) antigen, there was a decrease in released virus [6]; however, although the interferon-induced inhibition of assembly seemed to result in a relatively small decrease in the number of virus particles released, there was a marked inhibition in the infectivity of the MLV particles produced in one AKR-MLV system [6]. This observation has been confirmed in both chronic and acute Moloney MLV infection in TB cells [11]. It would seem, therefore, that, although in some systems interferon treatment resulted in marked inhibition of virus release, in others, particle production was almost normal, but the virus released was quite deficient in infectivity [1].

One possible basis for the low infectivity of the MLV produced by interferon-treated TB cells was a decrease in the amount of viral envelope glycoprotein gp69/71 associated with the virions. This conclusion was based on the reduced molar ratio of gp69/71 relative to other structural proteins in ^{35}S-methionine-labeled defective particles, as well as the reduced amount of ^{3}H-glucosamine incorporated into the glycoprotein (gp69/71) of these virions. The deficiency in gp69/71 may account for part, if not all, of the decrease in infectivity of these particles, since it has been shown that gp69/71 is responsible for the recognition and binding of the virion to the receptor sites on the cell membrane [12].

Apart from its antiviral activity, IFN has been shown to alter cellular parameters, in particular, those involved in cell growth. There may be a correlation between this property of interferons, termed the anticellular activity, and their antiviral activity since cells which respond to the anticellular activity of interferons also appear to be sensitive to the anti-lytic virus effect [14]. It is not clear, however, whether similar correlations exist between the interferon-induced inhibition of MLV production and the anticellular or anti-lytic virus activities of interferons. One could argue for instance, that the inhibition of MLV is mediated through the anticellular effect since production of MLV has been shown to be affected by the cell cycle [15] and extends both the G_1 and $S+G_2$ phases [16, 17, 18].

In comparing the anti-MLV, anti-EMC virus and anti-cellular activities of interferons, we have used three parameters for measuring the anti-cellular effects: inhibition of (i) cell division; (ii) DNA synthesis; or, (III) ornithine decarboxylase (ODC) induction. Inhibition of ODC induction has been shown to be an independent parameter for the anticellular activity of interferons [19, 20]. Indeed, the anti-

Table I. Effects of interferon on virus production in two Swiss 3T3-sublines, D-8 and H-2

		Concentration of interferon (U/ml)			
		10	25	50	100
Inhibition of:					
MLV (%)[a]	D-8	70	85	90	100
	H-2	65	95	95	100
EMC (log_{10})[b]	D-8	0	not done	1.0	1.0
	H-2	0.7	not done	4.8	4.8

[a] Subconfluent cultures of M-MuLV-infected cells, D-8 and H-2 (1×10^5 cells per 100 mm petri dish in 10 ml of Dulbecco modified Eagles' medium containing 10% fetal calf serum) were incubated for 24 h with L-cell interferon (specific activity 2×10^7 units per mg protein). Culture fluids were replaced with fresh medium containing interferon and after 24 h, MLV released into culture fluids was measured by assay of reverse transcriptase activity. Fluids were clarified by low speed centrifugation and virus was pelleted by sedimentation for 1 h at $105{,}000 \times g$. Pellets were resuspended in 100 ul of 20 mM Tris HCl pH 7.5, 100 mM NaCl, and 1 mM EDTA. Reverse transcriptase activity in the virus pellet was determined by incorporation of ^{3}H-TMP in the presence of poly A oligo dT template primer. Since cell number changed with the interferon concentration, results were corrected for original fluid volume and cell number at time of harvest. MLV from control cultures of D-8 and H-2 without interferon (100% activity) catalyzed the incorporation of 0.27 and 0.53 pmoles ^{3}H-TMP per min respectively.

[b] Parallel cultures of D-8 and H-2 were infected with EMC virus (MOI of 0.1) after 24 h treatment with interferon. After an additional 24 h, fluids were harvested; clarified by low speed centrifugation; and EMC virus was titered by infecting L-cells in 96-well microtiter plates with serial virus dilutions. CPE was recorded at 24 and 48 h post-infection. Results are given as inhibition of virus growth in log_{10}.

MLV effect of interferons can be dissociated from both its anticellular and antiviral activities. This was shown in the following manner: Swiss 3T3-cells, susceptible to the anticellular and antiviral effects of mouse interferon, were infected with Moloney-MLV at a multiplicity of one. The chronically infected cells were cloned by plating in a microtiter dish. Two of the clones were tested for susceptibility to interferon by assaying three parameters: (i) anti-MLV effect; (ii) anti-EMC virus activity and (iii) anticellular effects. Table I shows a dose-response effect of interferons on the production of MLV in two cell clones, D-8 and H-2. The virus released into the medium was assayed for reverse transcriptase activity and activity was corrected for cell number in the cultures. The sensitivity of the clones was similar. Virus production was also monitored by focus formation on S^+L^--cells [21] and parallel reduction curves were obtained (results not shown), indicating that the residual virus released from IFN-treated cells was fully infectious. In contrast to the anti-MLV effect, EMC virus was inhibited by interferon differentially in D-8 and H-2 cells; 50 U/ml reduced EMC virus yield by over 4 logs in H-2 but only 1 log in D-8 cells.

Next, the anticellular effects curve of interferon on: (i) cell division; (ii) DNA synthesis, as measured by thymidine incorporation; and, (iii) induction of ornithine decarboxylase (ODC) enzyme activity. All of the above activities were inhibited (table II). Comparison of D-8 and H-2 sensitivities indicated that for D-8 cultures, the amount of interferon required for 50% reduction was about 5-fold more for cell number, 45-fold more for DNA synthesis, and 3-fold more for ODC activity, as compared to H-2 cultures. Thus, the H-2 subclone appeared to be more sensitive than the D-8 subclone in terms of both the anti-EMC virus and anticellular activities of interferon; however, MLV inhibition in the two subclones was similar. These results suggested that interferon may affect cell growth functions and EMC replication through pathways different from those by which MLV production is inhibited.

To test this hypothesis further, several additional cell lines were infected with Moloney-MLV and analyzed for their ability to develop antiviral states against EMC virus and MLV after interferon treatment. Of the cells tested, the results obtained with NIH-3T3 cells [22], chronically infected with MLV, were most intriguing. Table III demonstrates that 1500 u/ml of interferon inhibited MLV

Table II. Anticellular effects of interferon in D-8 or H-2 subclones

Growth parameter	Concentration of interferon (U/ml)		
	10	50	100
Cell number (%)[a]			
D-8	100	92	48
H-2	65	38	23
Ornithine decarboxylase[b] induction (%)			
D-8	100	71	52
H-2	63	40	37
^{3}H thymidine incorporation[c]			
D-8	91	52	45
H-2	45	11	8

[a] Inhibition of cell multiplication. Cultures were treated with interferon for 48 h as described in table II. After fluids were harvested for reverse transcriptase assay, the monolayers were trypsinized for determination of cell number. Control cultures of D-8 and H-2 without IFN (100%) gave cell counts of 3.2×10^5 and 6.5×10^5, respectively.

[b] Inhibition of ornithine decarboxylase (ODC) induction. Quiescent cultures were prepared by serum depletion The cultures were stimulated with 10% serum in the presence of increasing concentrations of interferon and ODC activity in the cells was measured at the end of 6 h following serum addition. Values are expressed as percent of control cultures stimulated in the absence of interferon. The level of ODC activity in unstimulated cultures was less than 0.1 nmoles $^{14}CO_2$ released per mg cell protein per h. ODC activities in serum-stimulated D-8 and H-2 subclones were 2.58 and 2.26 nmoles $^{14}CO_2$/mg/h, respectively.

[c] Inhibition of DNA synthesis. The incorporation of ^{3}H-thymidine in quiescent cultures stimulated with serum was measured. After 30 h incubation, incorporation into acid-precipitable DNA was determined and is expressed as percent of control cultures which were stimulated in the absence of IFN. Quiescent and serum-stimulated D-8 cultures incorporated 5×10^5 cpm per culture while similar values for H-2 were 2×10^3 and 2.7×10^5 cpm per culture, respectively.

production by over 95%, while this high interferon concentration had no effect on EMC virus replication. Next, we tested the anticellular activity of interferon on these cells (NIH 3T3-MuLV). Interferon treatment had no inhibitory effects on cell division, DNA synthesis, or ODC enzyme induction. Similar resistance to interferon in terms of these parameters was also observed in NIH-3T3 cells not infected with MLV and obtained from a different source (results not shown). This cell line (NIH 3T3) thus showed a complete dissociation of the anti-MuLV activity from the anti-EMC or anticellular effects induced by interferons.

Table III. Effect of interferon on virus production in NIH-3T3 cells

	Concentration of interferon (U/ml)					
	0	10	30	500	1000	1500
Inhibition of[a]						
MLV (%)	0	60	75	80	85	90
EMC (%)	0	0	0	0	0	0

[a] Subconfluent NIH-3T3 cells, chronically infected with MLV, were incubated with interferon as described in table II. MLV production and EMCV replication in these cultures were assayed as described in table II. MLV production in control cultures without interferon (100% activity) catalyzed the incorporation of 1.16 pmoles ^{3}H-TMP per min. Inhibition of replication of EMCV and MLV are listed as percent inhibition.

The finding, that two subclones, isolated from a single culture of Swiss-3T3 cells chronically infected with MLV, exhibited different ranges of sensitivity to IFN which suggested variability among cells in a population. While variability was not observed with the anti-MLV activity, the clones differed in their sensitivities to both the anti-EMC virus and anticellular activities. Such a variability could have developed at one of two stages: (i) during cell passage; or, (ii) subsequent to infection by MLV. Since MLV infection of fibroblasts in a culture appears to have no effect on the cellular phenotype, the latter possibility is less likely.

Three different parameters were assayed for the anticellular effect of interferons; of the three, cell division appeared to be the most sensitive. This may be explained by the fact that interferons affect not only the G_1 and S phases (analyzed by ODC induction and DNA synthesis), but also the G_2 phase of the cell cycle [16]. In the two subclones D-8 and H-2, DNA synthesis was more sensitive to the inhibitory effect of interferon than induction of ODC. This is consistent with the observation that the inhibition of DNA synthesis in IFN-treated Swiss-3T3 cells is not a direct consequence of the inhibition of ODC induction [19].

Resistance of cells to interferons might be attributed to either a lack of receptors for interferon or to a deficiency in an intracellular factor required for establishment and/or maintenance of the antiviral and anticellular activities. NIH-3T3 cells appeared to be completely resistant to interferon in terms of the anti-EMC and anticellular activities, but they retained sensitivity to the anti-MLV activity. There are at least two possible explanations for the differential inhibitions of MLV and EMC virus in NIH-3T3 cells: (i) two different receptors for IFN are responsible for the establishment of antiviral states against EMC and MLV, and NIH-3T3 cells are devoid of the receptors necessary to initiate the anti-EMC viral state; or, (ii) there is only one type of receptor for interferon, but NIH-3T3 cells are deficient in an intracellular factor needed for the expression of the anti-EMC virus activity. Several enzymatic systems have been implicated in the anti-EMC viral state induced by interferons. One pathway involves induction of a synthetase activity which catalyzes the polymerization of 2'5'-oligo-A and this oligonucleotide induces a latent endonuclease activity in the interferon-treated cells [1]. Preliminary observations of *Epstein et al.* (personal communication) have indicated that 2'5'-oligo-A synthetase is induced in the same NIH-3T3 cell line in which EMC-virus replication is not inhibited after interferon treatment. This observation suggested the existence of receptors for interferon for the initiation of what is thought to be an anti-EMC virus activity. Work in progress indicates this pathway in NIH-3T3 cells is aborted at a later step, the level of the 2'5'-oligo-A-dependent endonuclease. This enzyme is lacking in NIH-3T3 cells.

Finally, it has been shown that retroviruses as well as lytic viruses can be used for assaying the antiviral activity of interferons [23]. In view of the present results, use of the standard assays (e. g. EMC virus inhibition) may not be sufficient for the determination of cell sensitivity to interferons, since cells, resistant to the anti-lytic virus activity of interferons, may still respond to the anti-MLV effect.

We are also in the process of studying VSV produced by interferon-treated L-cells. We have so far observed that, in L-cells treated with 30 U of interferon/ml, there was an approximately 200-fold reduction in the titer of infectious VSV production; however, virus particle production, as measured by VSV particle-associated RNA, N-protein, or transcriptase was inhibited by a maximum of 10-fold by this concentration of interferon. In addition, there was biochemical and morphological evidence of a significant reduction in glycoprotein (G) and membrane protein (M) content of VSV particles released from interferon-treated cells. The results in some respects resemble those previously reported for interferon-treated TB-cells infected with MLV. We concluded, therefore, that such findings are not limited to murine RNA tumor virus systems [24].

When the effects of tunicamycin (TM), and inhibitor of glycosylation of proteins, and IFN on VSV released from mouse cells were compared, they were both found to reduce the production of infectious VSV by 80- to 100-fold; to decrease the amounts of G and M viral proteins in VSV released from IFN-treated cells; and to inhibit an early step in the formation of asparagine-linked oligosaccharide chains, so that the incorporation by membrane preparations from interferon-treated cells of N-acetylglucosamine into glycolipid with the properties of dolichol derivatives was inhibited. It is possible that this effect of interferon-treatment is related to the deficiency in glycosylation of MLV and VSV protein, but there is as yet no biological data linking these findings [25].

The inhibition of some membrane-associated viruses by treatment with relatively moderate concentrations of interferon may be a widespread phenomenon that is closely related to functional abnormalities in the proteins incorporated into noninfectious virions produced by such cells. Since many studies have demonstrated that VSV particles with reduced amounts of glycoprotein are low in infectivity, it is likely that at least some of the reduced infectivity of VSV particles, produced by interferon-treated cells, was due to the reduced amount of this protein incorporated into such particles. It is possible that induced changes, that have been reported to occur in the plasma membrane of interferon-treated cells, may account for the alterations in infectivity of both VSV and murine RNA tumor viruses, since these viruses bud from the cell surface as a terminal step in the replication process [26].

Acknowledgments

The work done at Georgetown University was supported by American Cancer Society Grant # CD-56.

A. P. acknowledges the support of the Stiftung Volkswagenwerk. The authors thank *Joan Mok* for typing of the manuscript.

References

1 Friedman, R. M.: Antiviral activity of interferons. Bact. Rev. *41:* 543 (1977).
2 Strauchen, J. A.; Young, N. A.; Friedman, R. M.: Interferon-mediated inhibition of mouse mammary tumor virus expression in cultured cells. Virology *82:* 232 (1977).

3 Sen, G. C.; Sarkar, N.: Effects of interferon on the production of murine mammary tumor virus by mammary tumor cells in culture. Virology *102:*431 (1980).
4 Billiau, A.; Sobis, H.; De Somer, P.: Influence of interferon on virus-particle formation in different oncoRNA-virus cancer-cell lines. Int. J. Cancer *12:* 646 (1973).
5 Friedman, R. M.; Ramseur, J. M.: Inhibition of murine leukemia virus production in chronically infected AKR cells: A novel effect of interferon. Proc. natn. Acad. Sci. USA *71:*3542 (1974).
6 Pitha, P. A.; Rowe, W. R.; Oxman, M. N.: Effect of interferon on exogenous, endogenous, and chronic murine leukemia-virus infection. Virology *70:*324 (1976).
7 Shapiro, S. Z.; Strand, M.; Billiau, A.; Synthesis and cleavage processing of oncoRNA-virus proteins during inhibition of virus-particle release. Infect. Immunity *16:*742 (1977).
8 Billiau, A.; Heremans, H.; Allen, P. T.; De Maeyer-Guignard, J.; De Somer, P.: Trapping of oncoRNA-virus particles at the surface of interferon-treated cells. Virology *73:*537 (1976).
9 Chang, E.; Mims, S. J.; Triche, T. J.; Friedman, R. M.: Interferon inhibits mouse leukemia-virus release: An electron microscope study. J. gen. Virol. 34: 363 (1977).
10 Fan, H.; MacIsaac, P.: Virus-specific RNA synthesis in interferon-treated mouse cells productively infected with Moloney murine leukemia virus. J. Virol. *27:*449 (1978).
11 Chang, E. H.; Myers, M. W.; Wong, P. K. Y.; Friedman, R. M.: The inhibitory effect of interferon on a temperature-sensitive mutant of Moloney murine leukemia virus. Virology *77:* 99 (1977).
12 Friedman, R. M.; Maheshwari, R. K.; Jay, F. T.; Czarniecki, C. W.: Mechanism of interferon inhibition of viruses that bud from the plasma membrane. Ann. N. Y. Acad. Sci. *350:* 533 (1980).
13 Gresser, I.: On the varied biologic effect of interferon. Cell Immunol. *34:* 406 (1977).
14 Kuwata, T.; Fuse, A.; Morinaga, N.: Effect of interferon on cell and virus growth in transformed human cell lines. J. gen. Virol. *33:*7 (1976).
15 Panet, A.; Ceda, H.: Selective degradation of integrated murine leukemia virus proviral DNA by deoxyribonuclease. Cell *11:*933 (1977).
16 Balkwill, F.; Taylor-Papadimitriou, J.: Interferon affects both G_1 and $S+G_2$ in cells stimulated from quiescence to growth. Nature, Lond. *274:*798 (1978).
17 Creasey, A. A.; Bartholomew, J. C.; Merigan, T. C.: Role of G_0-G_1 arrest in the inhibition of tumor cell growth by interferon. Proc. natn. Acad. Sci. USA *77:* 1471 (1980).
18 Strander, H.; Einhorn, S.: Effect of human leukocyte interferon on the growth of human osteosarcoma cells in tissue culture. Int. J. Cancer *19:*468 (1977).
19 Sreevalsan, T.; Rozengurt, E.; Taylor-Papadimitriou, J.; Burchell, J.: Differential effect of interferon on DNA synthesis 2-deoxyglucose uptake, and ornithine decarboxylase activity in 3T3-cells stimulated by polypeptide growth factors and tumor promoters. J. cell Physiol. *104:* 1 (1980).
20 Sreevalsan, T.; Taylor-Papadimitriou, J.; Rozengurt, E.: Selective inhibition by interferon of serum-stimulated biochemical events in 3T3-cells. Biochem. biophys. Res. Commun. *87:*679 (1979).
21 Bassin, R. H.; Tuttle, N.; Fishinger, P. J.: Rapid cell culture assay techniques for murine leukemia viruses. Nature, Lond. *229:* 564 (1971).
22 Jainchill, J. L.; Aaronson, S. A.; Todaro, G. J.: Murine sarcoma and leukemia viruses: Assay using clonal lines of contact-inhibited mouse cells. J. Virol. *4:* 549 (1969).

23 Aboud, M.; Weiss, O.; Salzberg, S.: Rapid quantitation of interferon with chronically oncoRNA-virus-producing cells. infect. Immunity *13:*1626 (1976).
24 Maheshwari, R. K.; Jay, F. T.; Friedman, R. M.: Selective inhibition of glycoprotein and membrane protein content of vesicular stomatitis virus released by interferon-treated cells. Science *207:* 540 (1980).
25 Maheshwari, R. K.; Banerjee, D. K.; Waechter, C. J.; Olden, K.; Friedman, R. M.: Interferon treatment inhibits glycosylation of a virus protein. Nature, Lond. *287:* 454 (1980).
26 Friedman, R. M.: Interferons: Interaction with cell surfaces. Interferon *1:* 55 (1979).

R. M. Friedman, MD, Professor of Medicine, Laboratory of Exp. Pathology, NIAID, National Institute of Health, Building 4/Room 312, USA-Bethesda, MD 20205

Interferon Inhibits the Establishment of Fibroblast Infection by Avian Retroviruses

C. Jungwirth[1], *W. Strube*[1], *M. Strube*[1], *H. Kroath*[1], *T. Graf*[2]

[1] Institut für Virologie und Immunbiologie der Universität Würzburg Würzburg, FRG
[2] Institut für Virologie, Deutsches Krebsforschungszentrum Heidelberg, FRG

Introduction

Interferons inhibit the replication of cytocidal viruses and various tumor viruses. The inhibition of retrovirus replication so far studied occurs mainly late in the infectious cycle at the level of virus maturation or release [1]. All detailed studies on the mechanism of inhibition of retroviruses have been carried out with murine viruses. Information on the mechanism of inhibition of avian retroviruses by chicken interferon is scarce and apart from the inhibition of Rous sarcoma virus (RSV), measured by focus assay and tumor induction in chicken, no detailed study on the mode of action of homologous interferon has been reported [2, 3]. To extend previous studies on the mechanism of action of chicken interferon, we have studied the effect of interferon on transformation and replication of avian RNA tumor viruses.

Results and Discussion

Rous Sarcoma Virus-Induced Cell Transformation Is Inhibited by Chicken Interferon

As shown in figure 1, pretreatment of secondary chicken embryo fibroblasts (CEF) with doses of interferon as low as 16 units/ml, inhibited transformation of cells with RSV as determined by morphological inspection. In addition, virus titrations by focus formation

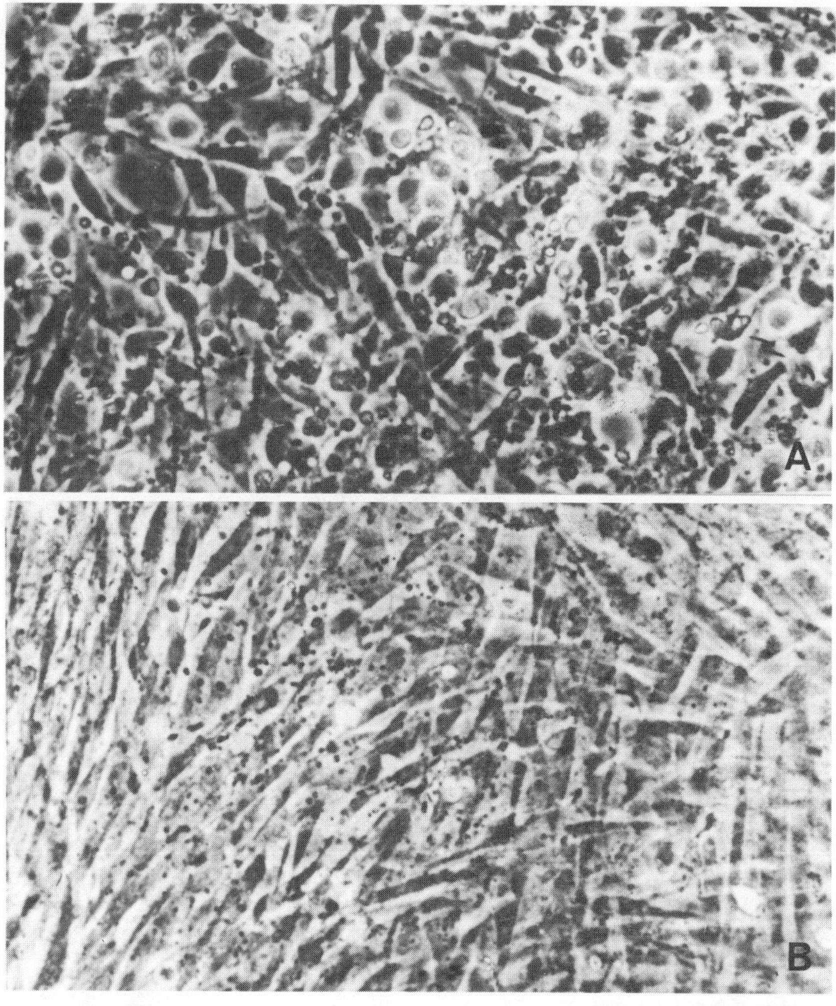

Figure 1. Inhibition of Rous sarcoma virus-specific cell transformation by interferon. Secondary CEF were seeded in 35 mm dishes at $3x10^5$ cells per dish in 2 ml of growth medium. Interferon (16 units/ml) was added and the cultures incubated for 20 h at 37°C. The cultures were infected with approximately $1x10^4$ PFU in 0,2 ml SR-RSV-D for 30 min. Fresh medium containing the same interferon dose was added. Two days later transformation was scored by phase-contrast microscopy and the supernatants were harvested for virus titrations.

(A) Control: Not treated with interferon.

(B) Cultures to which interferon (16 units/ml) were added 20 h before infection. The round refractile cells represent virus-transformed cells.

showed that pretreatment of cells with increasing doses of interferon resulted in a strong inhibition of focus-forming activity in the supernatant [4]. To decide whether the transformation process was inhibited by interferon or only secondary to an inhibition of viral replication, a CEF-cell strain, infected with a temperature-sensitive mutant RSV-TaSp7, was grown at 42° or 36°C [5]. Cultures from this cell strain were exposed to interferon doses up to 200 units/ml for 20 h and then shifted from non-permissive to permissive temperature and vice versa. It was found that, even at the highest interferon concentrations used, cell transformation was not inhibited. Therefore, it seems likely that the inhibition of transformation of chicken cells by RSV results from an inhibition of the viral infection. Further studies were carried out to determine the effect of interferon on the replicating ability of RSV. For this purpose a non-transforming mutant tdSR-RSV-D was used.

Replication of tdSR-RSV-D in Interferon-Treated Chicken Embryo Fibroblasts

The effect of homologous interferon was studied in de novo infected CEF and on an established infection of tdSR-RSV-D. The observed interferon effects on infectious virus in the cell supernatant, as determined by plaque assay, are summarized in table I. In exogenous infected CEF, even pretreated with only 20 units/ml of interferon, a reproducible inhibition of infectious virus formation could be detected. These results thus paralleled the response obtained with RSV-infected cells. In contrast, if homologous interferon at 10-fold higher concentrations (200 u/ml) was added to an established infection of tdSR-RSV-D for 20 h, the titers of infectious virus in the supernatant of control- and interferon-treated cells differed only marginally. Determining the interferon effect by metabolic labeling of extracellular virus particles or virus-associated reverse transcriptase activity also showed a more pronounced effect of interferon in freshly infected cells. These results support the notion that interferon has an inhibitory effect on the early phase of the RSV-replication cycle. Reduced interferon sensitivity of tdSR-RSV-D in a chronic infection does not result from the development of a general interferon resistance. To confirm this, tdSR-RSV-D-infected cells were superinfected with vesicu-

Table I. Interferon effects on formation of infectious tdSR-RSV-D in freshly infected or chronically infected chicken embryo fibroblasts. Conditions for plaque assay and preparation as well as assay of partially purified interferon have been described previously [4, 6]. Secondary CEF were treated for 18 h before infection with interferon at the indicated concentrations. Three days after infection, medium was harvested and after serial dilution, the RNA-tumor-virus titer was measured. To determine whether chicken interferon also effects established infections of tdSR-RSV-D, secondary CEF were infected at 5 PFU/cell and, after confluency, were reseeded into new petri dishes. On the third day, confluent cultures were reseeded and interferon was added at the indicated concentrations to some of the cultures. Two days later, the medium was changed and new interferon was added at the same concentration. After two further days, cells and medium were harvested and analyzed for formation of extracellular virus

	Freshly tdSR-RSV-D-infected cells		Chronically tdSR-RSV-D-infected cells	
Interferon u/ml	PFU/Plate	Inhibition %	PFU/Plate	Inhibition %
–	$3{,}2 \times 10^8$	0	$4{,}2 \times 10^8$	0
20	$6{,}0 \times 10^6$	98	–	–
50	$5{,}8 \times 10^6$	98	$3{,}1 \times 10^8$	79
100	$3{,}0 \times 10^6$	99	$2{,}2 \times 10^8$	52

lar stomatitis virus (VSV) and the effect of interferon was studied. As in normal CEF, it was found that low doses of interferon inhibited VSV-specific protein synthesis (fig. 2).

The striking inhibition of cell transformation and replication by RSV which is observed in chicken cells, pretreated with low concentrations of interferon before infection, confirms earlier reports which showed that focus formation by this virus is reduced by an interferon-like inhibitor [2]. The reported alterations of the replication cycle of tdSR-RSV-D by chicken interferon treatment differ in several respects from the interferon effects on the replication of murine retroviruses. The strong reduction of infectious virus particles by low doses of interferon is only observed when interferon is added before infection but not when added at even higher concentrations to fully infected cultures. On the other hand, effects of mouse interferon on the chronic infection of several murine onco-RNA viruses have been frequently reported [1]. Also, in contrast to some murine retroviruses, we have so far not found any alteration in the pattern of structural proteins between virus particles released from control- and interferon-treated cells.

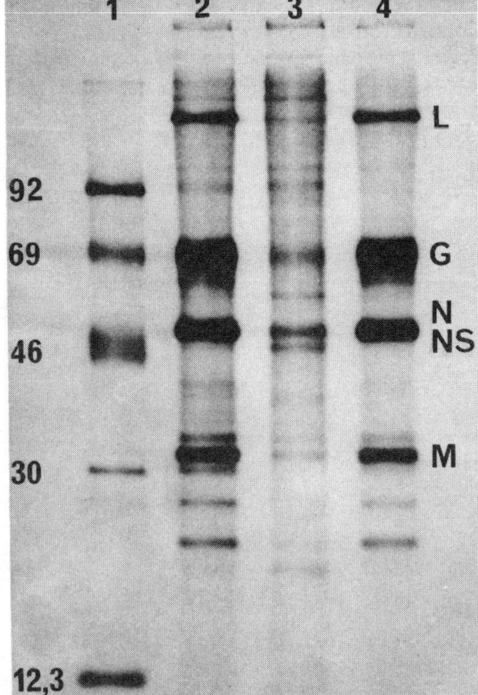

Figure 2. Inhibition of vesicular stomatitis virus-specific protein synthesis in tdSR-RSV-D-infected chicken cells. Chicken cells chronically infected with tdSR-RSV-D were treated with homologous interferon (100 u/ml) as described in table I. Four days after infection with tdSR-RSV-D, the chicken cells were superinfected with vesicular stomatitis virus (m.o.i. 20 PFU/cell); 4 h. p.i. the cells were labeled with 100 μCi ^{35}S-methionine (750 Ci/mMol) for 1 h. Cells were scraped from the petri dish and washed with cold phosphate-buffered saline. Cells were lysed and proteins were separated by PAG-electrophoresis on a 14,5% polyacrylamidegel [7].

Track 1: molecular weight markers. Track 2: tdSR-RSV-D- and VSV-infected cells. Track 3: tdSR-RSV-D, interferon-treated, and VSV-infected cells. Track 4: VSV-infected cells.

A further study of the interferon-induced alterations of the early phase of retrovirus infection should reveal the molecular basis of the replication inhibition of RSV by interferon.

References

1 Billiau, A.: Effect of interferon on RNA tumor viruses in the interferon system. Tex. Rep. Biol. Med. *35:* 406–419 (1977).

2 Bader, J.: Production of interferon by chicken embryo cells exposed to Rous sarcoma cirus. Virology *16:* 436–443 (1962).

3 Force, E. E.; Stewart, R. C.: Relationship of interferon-like inhibitor production to Rous sarcoma virus growth and tumor formation in chickens. J. Immun. *97:* 126–130 (1966).

4 Graf, T.: A plaque assay for avian RNA tumor viruses. Virology *50:* 567–578 (1972)

5 Beug, H.; Claviez, M.; Jokusch, B. M.; Graf, T.: Differential expression of Rous sarcoma virus-specific transformation parameters in enucleated cells. Cell *14:* 843–856 (1978).

6 Jungwirth, C.; Horak, I.; Bodo, G.; Lindner, J.; Schultze, G.: The synthesis of poxvirus-specific RNA in interferon-treated cells. Virology *48:* 59 – 70 (1972).

7 Laemmli, U. K.: Cleavage of structural proteins during assembly of the head of bacteriophage T_4. Nature *227:* 680 – 685 (1970).

Prof. Dr. Ch. Jungwirth, Institut für Virologie und Immunologie, Universität Würzburg, Versbacher Landstr. 7, D-8700 Würzburg

Pharmacological Properties of Human Alpha and Beta Interferons

Miguel A. Lucero[1], *Henri Magdelenat*[1], *Wolf H. Fridman*[1], *Pierre Pouillart*[1], *Claude Billardon*[2], *Alfons Billiau*[3], *Kari Cantell*[4], *Ernesto Falcoff*[2]

[1] Section Médicale et Hospitalière,
[2] Section de Biologie de l'Institut Curie (Groupe INSERM 196), Paris, France
[3] Rega Institute for Medical Research, Leuven, Belgium
[4] State Serum Institute, Helsinki, Finland

The use of interferon (IFN) as a therapeutic agent for tumor-bearing patients has gained considerable interest after reports demonstrated potent enhancing effects of IFN on the immunologic system. Thus, besides its direct effect on tumor cell multiplication [1], IFN may influence the host-tumor relationship by activating cells with potential antitumor activity such as natural-killer (NK) cells [2,3], killer (K) cells [3], or macrophages [4]. IFN also plays a role due to its capacity to modify the metabolism of certain molecules involved in immunologic functions, such as antigen receptors [5], histocompatibility antigens [6a, 6b, 7], or receptors for the Fc-fragment of immunoglobulins [8, 9].

Human IFN, in sufficient amounts to perform clinical trials, can be prepared in various ways. Fresh leukocytes [10] or cultured lymphoblastoid cells [11] upon infection with certain viruses, produce IFN consisting mainly of α-type molecules (Hu IFN-α) as defined by the International Committee on Interferon Nomenclature [12]. Cultured human fibroblast, after induction with double-stranded RNA, produce β-type IFN (Hu IFN-β) [13]. These two types of IFN differ in their chemical structure [14, 15] and pharmacological properties [21, 22]. They also differ in at least some biological properties, e.g. in their relative effects on the growth of cultured human cells [16], and in their dose-response curves in certain assay systems [17].

The purpose of the present study was to compare these two IFNs as to their effects on certain immunological parameters which can be used as biological markers to follow potential therapeutic effects.

In particular the following parameters were chosen:

(a) Serum levels of carcinoembryonic antigen (CEA), a non-specific marker of tumor proliferation.

(b) Serum levels or release by cultured cells of β_2-microglobulin, a molecule associated with the major histocompatibility complex (MHC) products.

(c) NK activity of circulating lymphocytes, i.e. spontaneous cytotoxic effect of lymphocytes, exerted on certain tumor-cell lines.

The effects of IFNs were studied both in vitro, by addition of IFN to cultured cells, or in vivo, by measuring the parameters in patients given i.m. injections.

Table I gives an overview of the results obtained in 10 patients divided into 3 experimental groups.

In the first group, single i.m. injections of 10^7 units of either leukocyte or fibroblast interferon were given to 5 patients with metastatic cancer. Each patient received two injections at an interval of 1 week, the first injection consisting of one type of interferon and the second of the other type. Blood samples were taken a few minutes before injection and also 1, 4, 9, 24, 35, 48, 72, and 96 h after injection. A second experimental group was treated similarly, except that each patient received consecutive injections of the *same* type of interferon. In the third group, the effect of different doses of interferon was studied. It is clear that leukocyte interferon was easily detectable in the serum of injected patients; with fibroblast interferon, serum titers of antiviral activity were much lower and sometimes undetectable. Single i.m. injection of leukocyte interferon (10^7 units) in patients resulted in measurable levels of antiviral activity in the serum for several hours, with peak values at 1 to 4 h varying between 80 and 500 units/ml. With fibroblast interferon at similar dosages, only very small amounts of antiviral activity were detected for only a very short period after injection. This confirms the previous findings of several authors who also found that leukocyte and fibroblast interferons had different pharmacokinetic behavior in both man [21, 22] and animals [20].

Table II shows the influence of interferon inoculation on NK-cell activity. It is clear that both fibroblast and leukocyte interferons

Table I. Interferon concentration in serum of patients given single i.m. injections of leukocyte or fibroblast IFN

Exptal. group	Patient				IFN treatment		Peak IFN concentration in serum (units/ml)	
	Code	Age	Sex	Diagnosis (a)	Preparation type (b)	Dose (units $\times 10^6$)	Leukocyte IFN	Fibroblast IFN
1	YAO	57	F	Breast cancer	Leukocyte	10	112	
					Fibroblast	10		< 32
	LEG	68	F	Kidney cancer	Fibroblast	10		32
					Leukocyte	10	82	
	EUV	50	M	Osteosarcoma	Leukocyte	10	500	
					Fibroblast	10		32
	VAL	59	M	Epithelioma of rectum	Fibroblast	10		32
					Leukocyte	10	225	
	PCI	67	F	Epithelioma of rectum	Leukocyte	10	96	
					Fibroblast	10		< 32
2	FAB	28	F	Ovarian cancer	Leukocyte	10	132	
					Leukocyte	10	316	
	PIC	52	M	Melanosarcoma	Fibroblast	10		52
					Fibroblast	10		114
3	PIA	57	F	Fibrosarcoma	Fibroblast	6		64
					Leukocyte	6	128	
	ICO	70	F	Breast cancer	Fibroblast	3		< 32
					Leukocyte	3	< 32	
	BCR	73	M	Squamous-cell carcinoma (upper respiratory and digestive tract)	Fibroblast	1		ND
					Leukocyte	1	ND	

(a) All patients were in metastatic phase of the disease.
(b) I.m. injection given in indicated sequence with a 1-week interval.

Table II. NK-cell activity in patients given single i.m. injections of leukocyte or fibroblast IFN

Exptal. group	Patient				IFN treatment		NK-cell activity (a) (%^{51}Cr release)	
	Code	Age	Sex	Diagnosis	Preparation type	Dose (units × 10^6)	0h	48h
1	YAO	57	F	Breast cancer	Leukocyte	10	4	46
					Fibroblast	10	<1	50
	LEG	68	F	Kidney cancer	Fibroblast	10	15	31
					Leukocyte	10	16	38
	EUV	50	M	Osteosarcoma	Leukocyte	10	6	61
					Fibroblast	10	19	46
	VAL	59	M	Epithelioma of rectum	Fibroblast	10	57	60
					Leukocyte	10	21	70
	PCI	67	F	Epithelioma of rectum	Leukocyte	10	24	65
					Fibroblast	10	15	65
2	FAB	28	F	Ovarian cancer	Leukocyte	10	34	89
					Leukocyte	10	35	91
	PIC	52	M	Melanosarcoma	Fibroblast	10	66	79
					Fibroblast	10	71	72
3	PIA	57	F	Fibrosarcoma	Fibroblast	6	34	58
					Leukocyte	6	33	62
	ICO	70	F	Breast cancer	Fibroblast	3	26	53
					Leukocyte	3	49	59
	BCR	73	M	Squamous-cell carcinoma (upper respiratory and digestive tract)	Fibroblast	1	43	42
					Leukocyte	1	52	51

(a) Effector target cell ratio: 100/1

induced an increase in NK-cell activity. From the data of group 3 it can be seen that the threshold dose required to obtain this effect was similar ($3x10^6$ units) for both interferon preparations.

Both interferons have been shown by other authors to activate NK-cell activity when added to cultures of peripheral blood lymphocytes in vitro [4, 18]. It has also been shown by others [23] that i.m. injections of leukocyte interferon in patients were found to enhance NK-cell activity, detectable by testing the spontaneous cytotoxicity of the patients' peripheral lymphocytes towards tumor cells in vitro. These results were confirmed in the present study. Surprisingly, despite the low or undetectable serum levels of antiviral activity obtained, we also found that i.m. injections of fibroblast interferon were able to activate the NK-cell system in vivo to about the same extent as in patients treated with leukocyte interferon. Significantly, in a dose-response experiment it was found that the threshold dose to obtain activation of the NK-cell system in patients was about $3x10^6$ units for both types of interferon preparations. Therefore, previous interpretations of the low blood levels obtained with i.m. injections of fibroblast interferon as being due to destruction at the site of injection may have been premature. It is of interest to note that in patients with an initial high level of NK-cell activity, the effect of interferon was nil or negligible, suggesting either that in these patients most cells with NK-activity were already maximally active or that no further recruitment or maturation could be induced by interferon. In general, our experiments and those of others seem to indicate that fibroblast and leukocyte interferons have similar effects on the NK-cell system in vitro as well as in vivo [4, 18]. This is of particular significance as it is believed that activation of the NK-cell system is an important mechanism of the antitumor action of all interferons.

In contrast to what was seen in the NK-cell system, leukocyte and fibroblast interferons differed from each other in their effects on the release of β_2-microglobulin. This is shown in table III. It is evident that injections of leukocyte interferon were followed by an increase in circulating β_2-microglobulin. This was not the case for fibroblast interferon.

This difference may have been due to the variable amounts of interferon reaching the cells that produce β_2-microglobulin. Alternatively, it may be due to differential tissue specificity, or to inherently different capacities of leukocyte and fibroblast interferons to affect the

Table III. β_2-microglobulin level in serum of patients given i.m. injections of leukocyte or fibroblast IFN

Exptal. group	Patient				IFN treatment		β_2-microglobulin level in serum			
							mg/l at:		% increase	
	Code	Age	Sex	Diagnosis	Preparation type	Dose (units $\times 10^6$)	0h	24h	Leucocyte IFN	Fibroblast IFN
1	YAO	57	F	Breast cancer	Leukocyte	10	2.7	4.5	67	
					Fibroblast	10	2.7	2.2		–19
	LEG	68	F	Kidney cancer	Fibroblast	10	3.1	4.1		32
					Leukocyte	10	3.2	6.1	91	
	EUV	50	M	Osteosarcoma	Leukocyte	10	2.4	4.7	96	
					Fibroblast	10	2.4	2.5		4
	VAL	59	M	Epithelioma of rectum	Fibroblast	10	2.1	1.9		–10
					Leukocyte	10	2.3	3.3	43	
	PCI	67	F	Epithelioma of rectum	Leukocyte	10	3.8	5.4	42	
					Fibroblast	10	3.4	3.2		–6
2	FAB	28	F	Ovarian cancer	Leukocyte	10	1.9	3.8	100	
					Leukocyte	10	2.0	3.7	95	
	PIC	52	M	Melanosarcoma	Fibroblast	10	1.6	2.0		25
					Fibroblast	10	1.5	1.8		12
3	PIA	57	F	Fibrosarcoma	Fibroblast	6	2.0	2.0		0
					Leukocyte	6	2.8	4.0	43	
	ICO	70	F	Breast cancer	Fibroblast	3	3.7	3.7		0
					Leukocyte	3	2.5	3.9	56	
	BCR	73	M	Squamous-cell carcinoma (upper respiratory and digestive tract)	Fibroblast	1	ND	ND		–
					Leukocyte	1	ND	ND		

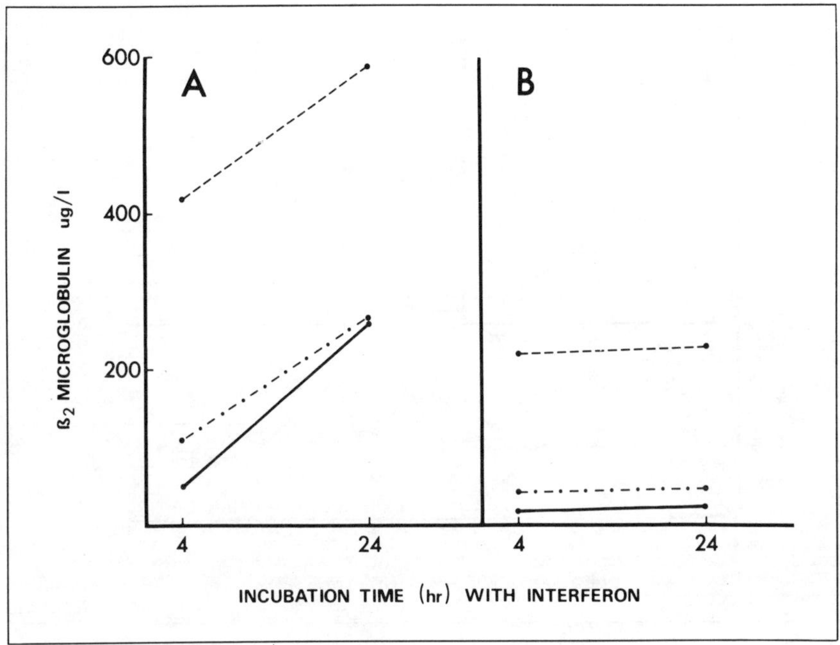

Figure 1. Release of β_2-microglobulin by lymphocytes (A) and fibroblasts (B) incubated with leukocyte or fibroblast IFN. Suspensions of lymphocytes (5x10^6 cells) or monolayers of fibroblasts (2.5x10^6 cells) incubated in 1 ml of control medium (● – – ●) or medium with 10^4 units of leukocyte (● – – –) or fibroblast (● – · – · – ●) IFN.

β_2-microglobulin system. In order to distinguish among these possibilities, in vitro experiments were performed and the results are shown in figure 1.

In this experiment suspensions of peripheral blood lymphocytes or monolayers of cultured fibroblasts were incubated at 37°C with 10^4 units/ml of either leukocyte or fibroblast interferon. Supernatant fluid samples were collected at 4 and 24 h and β_2-microglobulin contents were measured. All lymphocyte cultures (fig. 1A), including untreated controls, released measurable quantities of β_2-microglobulin. Fibroblast interferon had no effect on this spontaneous release. By contrast, cultures treated with leukocyte interferon released about 3 times more than the untreated controls, both at 4 and 24 h. A rather similar situation was encountered with fibroblast cultures (fig. 1B) with the difference that, in this case, β_2-microglobulin production was

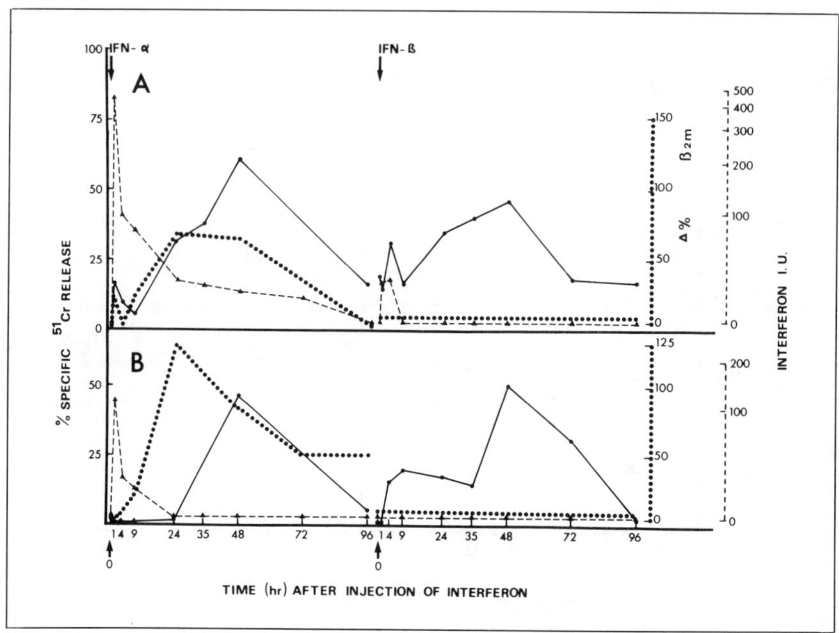

Figure 2. Serum levels of IFN (● – – – – ●), β_2-microglobulin (● · · · · · ·) and NK-cell activity (● ———— ●) in two patients (YAO and EUV) given a single i.m. injection of 10^7 units of leukocyte IFN, followed one week later by a same dose of fibroblast IFN.

very low in the cell supernatants of control and fibroblast interferon-treated cultures, whereas leukocyte interferon enhanced the release of β_2-microglobulin.

We can conclude that leukocyte interferon induced increased β_2-microglobulin release by lymphocytes and fibroblasts, while fibroblast interferon failed to do so. Therefore, the differential effect cannot be attributed to a different concentration of leukocyte or fibroblast interferons since, in the in vitro experiment, the cells were treated with the same amount. Nor can it be attributed to tissue specificity of interferon, since leukocyte interferon enhanced β_2-microglobulin release in both lymphocytes and fibroblasts. We are thus left with the hypothesis that the differential effects reflect distinct properties of leukocyte and fibroblast interferon preparations.

In the experiment, represented in figure 2, the kinetics of interferonemia, NK-activity, and β_2-microglobulin are summarized.

This figure shows two representative cases in which patients were first given an i.m. injection of 10^7 units of leukocyte interferon and a week later, the same dose of fibroblast interferon. It appears that both interferons enhanced NK-cell activity with similar kinetics, namely a small peak immediately after interferon administration and the maximum was reached 48 h after injection. After this maximum, NK-cell activity decreased after 96 h to the initial level. By contrast, the two interferons differed with respect to the levels of serum antiviral activity and β_2-microglobulin. Leukocyte interferon administration was followed by a peak of antiviral activity in the first hours after injection with a maximum after 4 h, and by an increase in serum β_2-microglobulin (over 100% of the initial level) peaking after 24 h; both parameters returned to initial level thereafter. Administration of fibroblast interferon was followed by low or undetectable antiviral activity in the serum.

As another parameter of possible effects of interferon on the tumor-host relationship, the serum levels of carcinoembryonic antigen were studied. The results of these determinations are summarized in table IV. No modifications related to interferon therapy were observed, regardless of whether pretreatment levels were high, low, or undetectable.

The enhanced release of β_2-microglobulin into the sera of patients treated with leukocyte interferon and in the supernatants of cells treated with the same interferon preparation may reflect enhanced synthesis or shedding of β_2-microglobulin. To ensure this point, it is necessary to verify that the observed effects on β_2-microglobulin release are really due to the IFN molecules and not to contaminants in the preparations. *Fellows et al.* (to be published), using pure human leukocyte IFN, have shown an increased release of β_2-microglobulin by the IFN-sensitive lymphoblastoid cell line, RAMOS, but not by the IFN-resistant cell line, NAMALVA. This observation favors the interpretation that the effects on β_2-microglobulin release are truly IFN-mediated.

Preliminary experiments indicate that both leukocyte and fibroblast interferons cause an increase in the amount of membrane β_2-microglobulin in lymphocytes and fibroblasts, although only leukocyte interferon enhances the release. It is therefore probable that both enhanced synthesis and enhanced shedding are involved in this phenomenon. β_2-Microglobulin is linked to the product of the major

Table IV. Serum levels of CEA (µg/l) in interferon-treated patients

Patients[1]	Hours after 1st injection of IFN									Hours after 2nd injection of IFN								
	0	1	4	9	24	35	48	72	96	0	1	4	9	24	35	48	72	96
YAD	24	35	24	36	19	ND	30	ND	29	31	43	31	34	99	39	24	24	23
LEG	0	0	0	0	0	0	0	0	0	0	0	0	0	0	0	0	0	0
EUV	0	0	0	0	0	0	0	0	0	0	0	0	0	0	0	0	0	0
VAL	5	8	5	5	10	5	6	5	8	0	6	0	14	0	0	0	0	7
PET	1170	1310	1350	1230	1150	1550	1330	1350	1470	1470	1870	1690	1875	1790	1860	1785	1880	2000
FAB	0	0	0	0	0	0	0	0	5	0	0	0	0	0	0	0	0	0
PIC	0	0	0	ND	0	ND	0	0	0	0	ND	ND	ND	0	ND	ND	ND	0
PIA	0	0	0	ND	0	0	0	0	0	0	ND	ND	ND	0	ND	ND	ND	0
TCH	0	0	0	ND	0	ND	0	0	0	0	ND	ND	ND	0	ND	ND	0	ND
BER	73	68	ND	89	66	ND	66	ND	78	74	76	ND	ND	81	ND	86	ND	64

[1] For specification of age, sex, diagnosis, and treatment schedule, see table I.

histocompatibility complex, which is HLA in humans [24] and H_2 in mice [25]. The products are themselves modified by, or associated with, the virus-coded [26] or tumor-associated antigens [27] which act as targets for cytotoxic T-lymphocytes [28]. It has been shown by others that the expression at the cell membrane of β_2-microglobulin as well as of H-2 and HLA molecules is increased when cells are incubated with interferon [6, 7]. Increased serum levels of β_2-microglobulin in patients treated with leukocyte interferon could then be due to enhanced expression of the major histocompatibility complex in various cells in the body. The importance of such a phenomenon in mediating the antitumor effect of interferon is still unknown. However, the different effects of leukocyte and fibroblast interferons on the metabolism of β_2-microglobulin or HLA molecules may result in different therapeutic effects in viral-infected or tumor-bearing patients.

Preparations of IFN have been shown to enhance the expression of various cell-membrane components such as receptors for synthetic polypeptides [29], receptor for concanavalin A [30], receptors for the Fc-fragment of IgG [8, 9] and also of CEA [31]. In the patients treated with IFN, no changes in serum levels of CEA were noted. Thus, it would appear that increased levels of β_2-microglobulin in patients treated with leukocyte interferon reflect a specific effect rather than just an unspecific increase in release of various cell-membrane components.

Acknowledgments

This work was supported by grants from INSERM (Institut National de la Santé et de la Recherche Médicale) (47-77-79, 78-4-082), DGRST (Délégation Générale à la Recherche Scientifique et Technique), Comité-Intersection of Curie Institute, and Cancer Research Foundation of the Belgian ASLK/CGER (General Savings and Retirement Fund).

We thank *Dr. M. Fellows* for providing K 562 cells, *Miss M. A. Provost, M. Rivière,* and *M. Thioux* for competent technical assistance.

References

1 Gresser, I.: On the varied biologic effects of interferon. Cell. Immunol. *34:* 406 (1977).

2 Gidlund, M.; Orn, A.; Wigzell, H.; Senik, A.; Gresser, I.: Enhanced NK-cell activity in mice injected with interferon and interferon inducers. Nature *273:* 759 (1978).

3 Herberman, R. B.; Djeu, J. Y.; Kay, H. D.; Ortaido, J. R.; Riccardi, C.; Bonnard, G. D.; Holden, H. T.; Fagnani, R.; Santoni, A.; Puccetti, P.: Natural-killer cells: Characteristics and regulation of activity. Immunol. Rev. *44:*43 (1979).

4 Herberman, R. B.; Ortaldo, J. R.; Bonnard, G. D.: Augmentation by interferon of human natural and antibody-dependent cell-mediated cytotoxicity. Nature *277:* 221 (1979).

5 Hamburg, S. I.; Marrejias, R. E.; Rabinovich, M.: Macrophage activation: Increased ingestion of igG-coated erythrocytes after administration of interferon inducers to mice J. exp. Med. *147:*593 (1978).

6a Lindahl, P.; Leary, P.; Gresser, I.: Enhancement of the expression of histocompatibility antigens of mouse lymphoid cells by interferon in vitro. Eur. J. Immunol. *4:*779 (1974).

6b Lindahl, P.; Gresser, I.; Leary, P.; Tovey, M. G.: Interferon treatment of mice: Enhanced expression of histocompatibility antigens on lymphoid cells. Proc. natn. Acad. Sci. USA *74:*1284 (1976).

7 Fellows, M.; Kamoun, M.; Gresser, I.; Bono, R.: Enhanced expression of HLA antigens and β_2-microglobulin on interferon-treated human lymphoid cells. Eur. J. Immunol. *9:*446 (1979).

8 Fridman, W. H.; Gresser, I.; Bandu, M. T.; Aguet, M.; Neauport-Sautes, C.: Interferon enhances the expression of Fc-γ-receptors. J. Immun. *124:*2436 (1980).

9 Itoh, K.; Inous, M.; Kataoka, S.; Kumagai, K.: Differential effect of interferon expression of igG- und igM-Fc receptors on human lymphocytes. J. Immun. *124;* 2589 (1980).

10 Cantell, K.; Hirvonen, S.: Large-scale production of human leucocyte interferon containing 10^8 units per ml. J. gen. Virol. *39:*541 (1978).

11 Strander, H.; Mogensen, K. E.; Cantell, K.: Production of human lymphoblastoid interferon. J. clin. Microbiol. *1:*116 (1975).

12 Stewart, W. E.: Interferon Nomenclature. Nature *286:*110 (1980).

13 Billiau, A.; van Damme, J.; van Leuven, F.; Edy, V. G.; de Ley, M.; Cassiman, J. J.; van den Bergher, H.; de Somer, P.: Human fibroblast interferon for clinical trials: Production, partial purification, and characterization. Antimicrob. Agents Chemother. *16:*49 (1979).

14 Knight, E. Jr.; Hunkapiller, M. W.; Korant, B. D.; Haroy, R. W. F.; Hood, L. E.: Human fibroblast interferon: Amino-acid analysis and amino-terminal amino-acid sequence. Science *207:*525 (1980).

15 Zoon, K. C.; Smith, M. E.; Bridgen, P. J.; Anfinsen, C. B.; Hunkapiller, M. W.; Hood, L. E.: Amino-terminal sequence of the major component of human lymphoblastoid interferon. Science *207:*527 (1980).

16 Einhorn, S.; Strander, H.: Is interferon tissue specific? Effect of human leukocyte and fibroblast interferons on the growth of lymphoblastoid and osteosarcoma cell lines. J. gen. Virol. *35:*573 (1977).

17 Edy, V. G.; Billiau, A.; de Somer, P.: Human fibroblast and leukocyte interferons show different dose-response curves in assay of cell protection. J. gen. Virol. *31:* 251 (1976).

18 Lucero, M. A.; Fridman, W. H.; Provost, M. A.; Billardon, C.; Pouillart, P.; Dumont, J.; Falcoff, E.: Effect of various interferons on the spontaneous cytotoxicity exerted by lymphocytes from normal and tumor-bearing patients. Cancer Res. *41:*294 (1981).

19 Cerottini, J. C.; Brunner, K. T.: In vitro assay of target cell lysis by sensitized lymphocytes. In: Bloom, Glade (eds.), In vitro methods in cell-mediated immunity, pp. 369–373 (Academic Press, New York 1971).

20 Edy, V. G.; Billiau, A.; de Somer, P.: Non-appearance of injected fibroblast interferon in the circulation. Lancet *i:*451 (1978).

21 Billiau, A.; de Somer, P.; Edy, V. G.; Clercq, E.; Heremans, H.: Human fibroblast interferon for clinical trials: Pharmacokinetics and tolerability in experimental animals and humans. Antimicrob. Agents Chemother. *16:*56 (1979).

22 Vilcek, J.; Sulea, I. T.; Zerebeckyj, I. L.; Yip, Y. K.: Pharmacokinetic properties of human fibroblast and leukocyte interferon in rabbits. J. clin. Microbiol. *11:*102 (1980).

23 Huddlestone, J. R.; Merigan, T. C.; Oldstone, M. B.: Induction and kinetics of natural killer cells in humans following interferon therapy. Nature *282:* 417 (1979).

24 Neauport-Sautes, C.; Bismuth, A.; Kourlisky, F. M.; Manuel, Y.: Relationship between HL-A antigens and β_2-microglobulin as studied by immunofluorescence on the lymphocyte membrane. J. exp. Med. *139:*55 (1974).

25 Vitetta, E. S.; Poulik, M. D.; Klein, J.; Uhr, J. W.: Beta 2-microglobulin is selectively associated with H-2 and TL alloantigens on murine lymphoid cells. J. exp. Med. *144:*179 (1976).

26 Senik, A.; Neauport-Sautes, C.: Association between H-2 and vaccine virus-induced antigens on the surface of infected cells. J. Immun. *122:*1461 (1979).

27 Meschini, A.; Invernizzi, G.; Parmiani, G.: Expression of alien H-2 specificities on a chemically-induced Balb/c fibrosarcoma. Int. J. Cancer *20:*271 (1977).

28 Zinkernagel, R. M.; Doherty, P. C.: MHC-restricted cytotoxic T-cells: Studies on the biological role of polymorphic major transplantation antigens determining T-cell restriction-specificity, function, and responsiveness. Adv. Immunol. *27:* 96 (1979).

29 Lonai, P.; Steinman, L.: Physiological regulation of antigen binding to T-cells; Role of a soluble macrophage factor and of interferon. Proc. natn. Acad. Sci. USA *75:*5662 (1977).

30 Huet, C.; Gresser, I.; Bandu, M. T.; Lindahl, P.: Increased binding of concanavalin-A to interferon-treated murine leukemia L-1210 cells. Proc. Soc. exp. Biol. Med. *147:*52 (1974).

31 Attallah, A. M.; Needy, C. F.; Noguchi, P. D.; Elisberg, B. L.: Enhancement of carcino-embryonic antigen expression by interferon. Int. J. Cancer *24:*49 (1979).

R. Falcoff, MD, Institut Curie, Section de Biologie, 26, rue d'Ulm, F-75231 Paris

Effect of Interferon on Certain Cellular Immune Functions

M. G. Masucci, E. Klein, G. Masucci, R. Szigeti, F. Vanky

Department of Tumor Biology, Karolinska Institute, Stockholm, Sweden

Introduction

Interferon (IFN) influences the immune system on several levels [8]. It abrogates mitogen- and antigen-induced blastogenesis of lymphocytes [1], suppresses antibody production [14] and delayed type hypersensitivity reactions [6 – 10]. On the other hand, it potentiates the phagocytic capacity of macrophages [7] and monocytes [13] and the cytotoxic potential of lymphocytes. IFN is produced during the interaction of sensitized lymphocytes with their targets [12] and also when lymphocytes are exposed to certain tumor cell lines [25]. The effect of IFN on cytotoxic systems is complex. It enhances the effector function while lowering the susceptibility of the targets [24].

We have studied the effect of IFN on: (1) the leukocyte migration inhibition (LMI) test which is considered to be an in vitro correlate of the delayed type hypersensitivity reaction [22]; (2) the cytotoxic activity exerted by unsensitized lymphocytes against certain tumor cell lines maintained in vitro. This effect is designated as natural killing (NK); (3) the cytotoxic activity exerted by lymphocytes of tumor-bearing patients against autologous and allogeneic tumor cells derived from surgical specimens.

Recently the genes which code for the synthesis of human leukocyte IFN have been transplanted into E. coli where they induced the production of polypeptides that have IFN activities as judged by biochemical, antiviral, and immunological evidences [18]. We have also tested the effect of the recombinant IFN in the LMI and the NK assays.

Results

Effect of IFN on the Leukocyte Migration Inhibition (LMI) Assay

The in vitro mobility of blood granulocytes can be measured quantitatively. It is inhibited by factors released by lymphocytes when they are exposed to mitogens or antigens to which they have been sensitized. We found that phytohemagglutinin- (PHA) and antigen-induced LMI was reduced in the presence of 100 U/ml IFN. In the PHA system the mean percentage inhibition decreased to 25% compared to 58% in the absence of IFN (table I). In the immune LMI system we used Epstein-Barr virus (EBV) antigens. The leukocyte migration of EBV seropositive individuals was inhibited by cell extracts from P3HR-1, an EBV genome positive cell line. This inhibitory effect was almost completely abolished in the presence of lymphoblastoid as well as in E. coli-derived IFN.

The direct LMI system is complex: the cell population collected from the buffy coat contains the lymphocytes which produce the leukocyte migration inhibitory factor (LIF) and also the migrating granulocytes upon which the factor acts. Our experiments, which aimed to

Table I. Effect of IFN on mitogen- and antigen-induced leukocyte migration inhibition[1]

Mitogen-induced	% MI	Antigen-induced	% MI
PHA	58	P3HR-1	43
PHA-ce	55	P3HR-1-ce	42
PHA-IFN	25	P3HR-1-IFN	12
PHA-IFNc	17	P3HR-1-IFNc	10

[1] The agarose microdroplet technique [17] was used. The migration areas were measured and the % migration inhibition (MI) calculated according to the formula

$$\% \text{ MI} = \frac{\text{mean migration area with antigen}}{\text{mean migration area without antigen}} \times 100$$

MI is considered positive when the % inhibition exceeds 20 in the antigen-induced system and 50 with PHA. Purified PHA (Wellcome) was added at a concentration of 1 μg/ml. Crude extract of the EBV-producer P3HR-1 line was used at a protein concentration of 50 μg/ml. 100 U/ml of IFN-alpha 1 (E.coli produced) (IFNc) [18] or lymphoblastoid IFN produced by the Namalwa cell line (IFN) [3] or E.coli control extract (ce) (the same amount of protein as in IFNc) were added where indicated.

Table II. Effect of IFN on the granulocyte migration inhibition induced by lymphokine containing PHA supernatant[1]

−IFN	+IFN[1]	+30 min IFN pretreatment	+IFN 30 min posttreatment
42.5 ±1.9	18.3 ±2.7	20.1 ±1.5	39.1 ±2.6

[1] The results represent the mean and SD of 10 experiments. The lymphokine was produced as described in table III.
[2] 100 U/ml of IFN were present during the migration period.

Table III. Effect of IFN on lymphokine production of lymphocytes induced by exposure to PHA[1]

−IFN	+IFN[1]	+IFN +anti-IFN
44 ±3.1	16.8 ±5.6	37.3 ±4.3

[1] The results represent the mean and SD of 4 experiments.
[2] The cells were incubated for 30 min with 100 U/ml IFN with or without simultaneous addition of anti-(100 U/ml) IFN serum, then washed thoroughly with medium and stimulated for lymphokine production with 1 μg/ml PHA. The values represent the % MI induced on separated granulocytes by the supernatants produced under various culture conditions.

reveal the mechanism of IFN action, suggested that IFN influences both components. The migration of separated granulocytes was tested by the indirect method with lymphokines derived from PHA-stimulated lymphocyte cultures (table II). The migration inhibition in this system was abrogated by the presence of 100 U/ml of IFN during the migration period. Furthermore, 30 min incubation of the granulocytes with IFN before addition of the lymphokine-containing material had the same effect while IFN did not affect the migration when it was added after the exposure to the lymphokine.

The effect of IFN on the LIF production by lymphocytes was tested as follows:

Lymphocytes were incubated with IFN (one sample also in presence of anti-IFN serum) washed and exposed to PHA (table III). The supernatants of PHA-treated lymphocytes were assayed for inhibition of migration of separated granulocytes. Preincubation with 100 U IFN/ml reduced LIF production. The lymphokine produced by the PHA-treated lymphocytes caused 44% MI while the corresponding material derived from IFN-pretreated lymphocytes caused only 16.7% MI. The IFN-induced suppression of LIF production was prevented by the simultaneous addition of anti-IFN serum.

Effect of IFN on Spontaneous Cytotoxicity against in Vitro Cultured Cell Lines

The NK phenomenon is defined operationally as the cytolytic potential of lymphocytes derived from donors without known sensitization history against the targets. Short-term exposure of lymphocytes to IFN results in considerably enhanced cytotoxic activity [24]. We refer to the effect of such lymphocytes as IFN-activated killing (IAK). The mechanism by which IFN imposes the elevated function on the cells is not known. It occurs in vivo also since administration of IFN or IFN-inducing substances to experimental animals and man were shown to elevate NK activity of their spleen or blood lymphocytes [9].

The characteristics determining the degree of NK sensitivity of a given cell is unknown. Cell lines can be divided in three categories: (1) sensitive in short-term assays i.e. within the range of the effector/target ratios used where considerable target-cell damage occurs at low ratios; (2) sensitive only in long-term assays; (3) insensitive.

Certain cell lines which are not killed in short-term ^{51}Cr-release assay are affected when the interaction with the effector lymphocytes is prolonged. It is likely that IFN production in the cultures is responsible for the activation of the effectors. IFN is known to be produced during cocultivation of lymphocytes with tumor-cell lines and supernatants from such mixed cultures were shown to enhance the cytotoxic potential of fresh lymphocytes [12]. It was found that IFN-pretreated effectors can kill the low sensitive targets with the kinetics shown for the highly sensitive K562 [2, 16].

The short-term NK and IAK systems differ only in the technical aspects in that the latter involves pretreatment of the effector cells. The two systems overlap, however, because lymphocytes of an individual exhibit high activity functions similar to the weakly active lymphocytes of another donor after in vitro exposure to IFN (fig. 1). Thus what can be achieved artificially with the lymphocytes of one individual can be a genuine level for another. The reason for the dif-

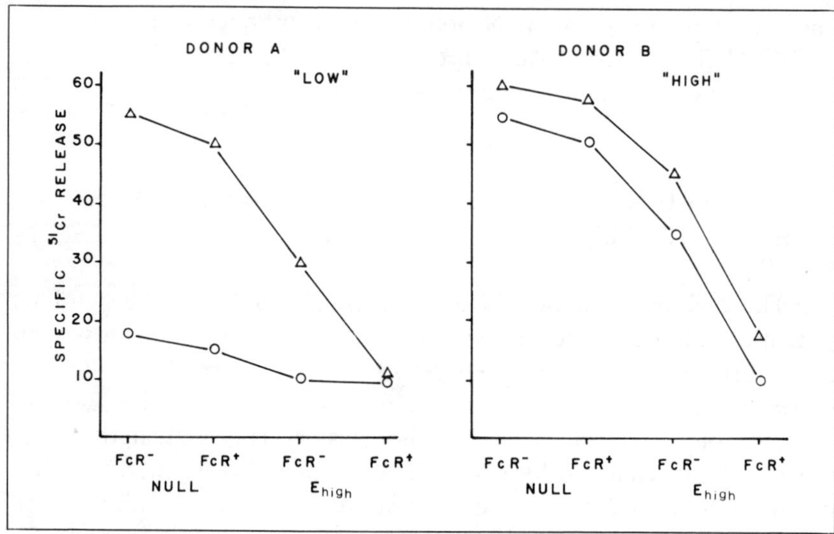

Fig. 1. Cytotoxic activity profile of blood lymphocytes separated from two individuals. Blood lymphocytes from two donors, one with high (A) and one with low (B) spontaneous cytotoxic activity against K562 were separated according to nylon adherence, E- and EA-rosetting capacity using the protocol described in *Masucci et al.* [15]. The results obtained with 4 subsets of the nylon-passed population are presented. These were the operational „null" and high avidity E-receptor subsets with or without concommittant expression of Fc-receptors. ^{51}Cr-release assay and IFN pretreatment of the effectors were performed as described in table IV. Effector target ratio 25:1.

ferent levels of activity in various individuals is unknown. Tumor patients have been found to have relatively low activity though this is not an absolute rule. Whether the patients belonged to the high or low NK categories did not relate to the clinical status. Low NK-active tumor patients' lymphocytes could be enhanced by IFN showing that the potentially active cells were not absent [26].

The effect of IFN is prompt but the expression of the activated state requires a few hours. The activated state decays with a half life of about 10 h [2, 16].

Saksela et al. [20] suggested that the mechanism, which leads to a higher number of targets killed by IFN-pretreated lymphocytes, is a recruitment of prekiller cells. They induced anti-K562 activity in a cell population which was depleted of NK effect by adherence to fibroblast monolayers. *Targan* and *Dorey* [23], using an assay which estimates the number of active killer cells, concluded also that IFN

Table IV. Cytotoxic activity of IFN-treated lymphocytes against targets of low and high NK sensitivity[1]

Effector/Target ratio	K562			Daudi		
	−IFN	+IFN[2]	ON	−IFN	+IFN[2]	ON
12 : 1	38	40	40	5	38	25
4 : 1	20	30	32	2	28	20
1.3 : 1	17	18	16	0	16	12
0.4 : 1	1	8	6	0	7	5

[1] Untreated and IFN-exposed lymphocytes were aliquoted into the wells of a V-shape microtiter plate (Falcon) in 150 μl volume. 20 μl of the ^{51}Cr-labeled target-cell suspension were delivered into each well. After 4 or 18 h (ON) incubation (at 37°C in a 5% CO_2 incubator), the radioactivity present in the cell-free supernatant was measured. The percentage specific lysis (% S) was calculated according to the following formula:

$$\% S = \frac{\text{release in the test} - \text{spontaneous release}}{\text{total release} - \text{spontaneous release}} \times 100$$

[2] Preincubated for 3 h in the presence of 1000 U/ml of lymphoblastoid IFN. The cells were washed before use as effectors.

treatment recruited new effectors. They showed in addition, however, that the lytic function of already active cells was enhanced.

It has been shown that the IFN-induced potentiation of killer function acts on the same lymphocyte subset which exert the spontaneous NK activity [15]. This fact and the observation that the boosting effect of IFN is more obvious with target of low NK sensitivity and that IFN-treated effectors kill a high and a low NK sensitive cell (K562 and Daudi) with similar efficiency (table IV) led us to formulate the following hypothesis: There is a heterogeneity in the lymphocyte population with regard to the expression of the lytic function. The thresholds of the lytic function for which various cell lines are sensitive differ. The differences in the dose-response curves with different targets reflect the proportion of cells reaching these thresholds. We assume that IFN elevates the lytic function temporarily. Consequently, IFN-treated cells will also affect targets whose sensitivity threshold is relatively high and are thus damaged only by lymphocytes expressing strong activity. Due to the different sensitivity of each target, the pre-killer designation is not absolute but characteristic for the particular system. Cells, defined as prekillers in one target system, may be killers when a more sensitive cell is used as target.

Effect of IFN on the Cytotoxic Activity against Freshly Separated Tumor Biopsy Cells

In experiments performed in search of antitumor reactivity in man we found that freshly harvested tumor cells from human sarcomas and carcinomas lack or possess low NK sensitivity. They were lysed by healthy donor's lymphocytes only when these belonged to the category of very high NK potential as indicated by strong effect on K562 cells. However, cytotoxicity could be induced against allogeneic tumor biopsy cells in 50% of the cases by incubating the lymphocytes for 2 – 3 h with IFN prior to the test [26]. Similar results on leukemias were reported by *Zarling et al.* [28]. Thus IFN did not induce cytotoxicity against autologous tumor cells. Such activity occurred with untreated lymphocytes in about 25% of the solid tumor cases tested, however IFN did not elevate its strength and, when it was absent, IFN did not induce it. Our interpretation was that the biopsy cells were killed by alloreactive cells triggered by IFN for the lytic function. The activation of cytotoxic precursors by IFN and the manifestation of cytotoxicity toward cells that carry alien histocompatibility antigens is similar to the finding with mitogen-activated murine cells [5].

This interpretation was substantiated by cold-target competition experiments which showed that when targets from surgical specimens, obtained from different donors, were killed by lymphocytes from one donor, different subpopulations, probably representing different alloreactive clones, caused the observed lysis (table V).

Table V. Summary of cold target competition tests in lytic systems against tumor biopsy cells with IFN-treated allogeneic lymphocytes as effectors[1]

			Ratio labeled : Unlabeled target		
	Competitor	No of tests	2 : 1	1 : 1	1 : 10
Biopsy	Non-identical	26	5[2]	22	35
	Identical	35	35	60	95

[1] The tumor cells were separated from surgical specimens [27]. Effector target ratio 50 : 1, 4 h ^{51}Cr-release assay. The lymphocytes were collected from healthy donors and from tumor patients.

[2] Mean % inhibition of cytotoxicity at the indicated ratios. The cytotoxic tests were performed as described in table IV.

Table VI. Generation of autotumor reactive killer cells in mixed cultures is inhibited by addition of IFN[1]

Effector cells cultured with[2]	IFN[3]	Target cells Autologous tumor cells		
	–	2/19[4]	10%[5]	7[6]
	+	1/12	8%	7
Autologous tumor cells	–	14/19	74%	33
	+	1/19	5%	5

[1] Results summarized from *Vanky* and *Argov*.
[2] Aliquots of T-cell-enriched nylon column-passed lymphocyte populations were mixed with tumor cells in plastic tissue culture flasks. The lymphocytes were also cultured alone. The cultures were incubated for 6 days at 37°C in a humidified atmosphere of 5% CO_2. After washing the cells were resuspended in medium and used as effectors in the cytotoxicity assays. Tumor cells were used directly after isolation from surgical specimens (sarcoma and carcinoma) as stimulators, frozen preserved during 6 days for the use as targets.
[3] 1000 U/ml IFN was added at the initiation of the cultures.
[4] Number of cases with cytotoxicity/total number of tests.
[5] Percentage of positive tests.
[6] Mean specific ^{51}Cr release in 4 h tests at 50 : 1 effector target ratio.

Effect of IFN on the Blastogeneic Response and Generation of Cytotoxicity against Autologous Tumor Biopsy Cells

In the human tumor system, the lack of IFN effect on the autologous cytotoxicity was puzzling. The obvious cause may habe been the absence or relatively low number of tumor-recognizing lymphocytes in a state of differentiation which responds to IFN. In a high proportion of cases, the blood lymphocytes of cancer patients have been shown to react with blast transformation and to develop killer cells against their own tumor cells after cocultivation in vitro [27]. These results suggest that lymphocytes, which recognize autologous tumor cells, are present in the blood. However, their number may not be sufficient to bring about detectable cytotoxicity. Cytotoxicity can be generated after an encounter with the antigen that triggers multiplication i.e. enlargement of the specific clone.

Addition of IFN to the autologous lymphocyte tumor cultures abrogated blastogenesis and the appearance of auto-tumor cytotoxicity (table VI). This can be explained by the inhibitory effect of IFN on

DNA synthesis, thereby counteracting the enlargement of the specific clone.

Discussion

It is likely that IFN plays an important regulatory role in the immune response. On the basis of the knowledge accumulated in various in vitro systems, the encounter between the antigen-carrying cell and the lymphocytes with the relevant receptor may cause the following events:

(a) *The recognition induces IFN production.* Interferon elevates the cytotoxic function of lymphocytes which are in a certain state of differentiation (null and low-avidity E-receptor-positive cells) and, consequently, a certain proportion of these reaches the threshold of activation required for the lysis. This threshold is dependent on the target-cell sensitivity. The activation is polyclonal and, therefore, those other than the specific antigen-carrying cells can also be killed i.e. transactivation occurs [21]. Whether the cytotoxicity can be detected depends on the number of lymphocytes which carry receptors to the antigens present on the target and the sensitivity of the target.

(b) *The recognition stimulates the lymphocytes to proliferation.* Part of these are in a differentiation state which does not express cytotoxic function (high-avidity E-receptor-forming cells). After some days the specific clone is enlarged and the lymphocytes are activated for cytotoxicity. Since the encounter with the same antigen will engage a larger proportion of cells in the reaction, the response will be amplified. Due to the larger number of specifically responsive cells, higher amounts of the activating factors (IFN or lymphokines) will be released.

Damage to the target which carries the antigen will be detectable, even if its cytotoxic sensitivity is relatively low. IFN may be an important factor in the control of these events, since antigen-induced enlargement of specific cytotoxic clones and the production of lymphokines are limited by IFN.

The versatility of the IFN effect on the immune system, including potentiation of certain effector functions together with its inhibitory effect on cell multiplication, has induced many investigations with the ultimate aim to assess its possible use for antitumor therapy. An important finding which motivated this direction was the elevated natural cytotoxic potential of lymphocytes imposed by IFN.

The view that natural cytotoxicity plays an important role in surveillance was based on the relatively high sensitivity of tumor-derived cell lines and the correlation between in vitro cytotoxic potential and in vivo rejection response when mouse strains were tested [11]. The demonstration of direct antitumor effects, obtained with certain cell lines, explains the enthusiasm for this postulated antitumor mechanism.

The low sensitivity of freshly harvested tumor cells (sarcoma, carcinoma, leukemia) to the cytotoxic effect of unmanipulated lymphocytes makes it improbable, however, that killer cells without immunological specificity have a surveillance function. It seems that tumor cells in vivo do not share the membrane properties of the in vitro model lines which exhibit high sensitivity to the genuine or activated killer cells without involving antigen-specific recognition.

On the other hand, the results obtained in allogeneic combinations indicate that, when sufficient numbers of the relevant antigen-recognizing cells are present in a differentiation state which conveys responsiveness to the activating effect of IFN, cytotoxicity can be manifested. In this context, it is important to emphasize that the proportion of lymphocytes which recognizes alloantigens is high [19].

In view of the results discussed in this paper on systems which reflect certain parameters of the immune response, the antitumor effect of IFN through immunological mechanisms seems to be limited. Apart from the enhancement of direct cytotoxicity, its effect was shown to be suppressive.

Due to the complexity of the immune system, the highly artificial in vitro conditions, in which its isolated components are tested, may not reflect the in vivo events. Our view is formulated and presented with the aim to provoke a caution in the expectations concerning the therapeutical antitumor effect of IFN.

Acknowledgments

This investigation was supported by PHS grant number 1 R01 CA 25184-01A1, awarded by the National Cancer Institute DHHS, and the Swedish Cancer Society.

Maria G. Masucci is supported by the Foundation Blancefort Boncompagni-Ludovisi född Bildt, Stockholm. *Robert Szigeti* is a recipient of a fellowship from the Swedish Institute, Stockholm.

References

1 Adams, A.; Strander, H.; Cantel, K.: Sensitivity of the Epstein-Barr virus transformed human lymphoid cell lines to interferon. J. gen. Virol. *28:* 207–217 (1975).

2 Berthold, W.; Masucci, M. G.; Klein, E.; Strander, H.: Interferon treatment elevates the cytotoxic potential of lymphocytes and thereby increases the frequency of functional killer cells (in press).

3 Bodo, G.: Production and purification of lymphoblastoid interferon. In: IKIS Acad. Sci. Acts. Proc. Symp. on Preparation, Standardization and Clinical Use of Interferon, pp. 49–57 (Zagreb, June, 1977).

4 Borecky, L.; Fuchsberg, N.; Zemla, J.; Lackovic, V.: Properties of the interferon-like virus inhibitor released during interaction of mouse-sensitized lymphocytes with their target cells. Eur. J. Immunol. *3:* 213–218 (1971).

5 Clark, W. R.: An antigen-specific component of lectin-mediated cytotoxicity. Cell. Immunol. *17:* 505–509 (1975).

6 De Mayer, E.; De Mayer-Giugnard, J.; Vandeputte, M.: Inhibition by interferon of delayed type hypersensitivity in the mouse. Proc. natn. Acad. Sci. USA *72:* 1753–1775 (1975).

7 Donahoe, R. M.; Huang, K. Y.: Interferon preparations enhance phagocytosis in vivo. Infection and Immunity *13:* 1250–1257 (1976).

8 Epstein, L.: Effects of interferon on the immune response in vitro and in vivo. In: Stewart, Interferons and their actions, pp. 91–132 (CRB Press, Cleveland, Ohio 1977).

9 Herberman, R.; Nunn, M.; Holden, H. T.; Staal, S.; Djeu, J.: Augmentation of natural cytotoxic reactivity of mouse lymphoid cells against syngeneic and allogeneic target cells. Int. J. Cancer *19:* 555–564 (1977).

10 Hirsch, M. S.; Ellis, D. A.; Black, P. H.: Immunosuppressive effects of an interferon preparation in vivo. Transplantation *17:* 234–236 (1974).

11 Kiessling, R.; Hochman, P. S.; Haller, O.; Shearer, G. M.; Wigzell, H.; Cudkowicz, G.: Evidence for a similar or common mechanism for natural killer-cell activity and resistance to hemopoetic grafts. Eur. J. Immunol. *7:* 655–663 (1977).

12 Koide, Y.; Takasugi, M.: Augmentation of human natural cell-mediated cytotoxicity by a soluble factor. I. Production of a N-cell-activating factor (NAF). J. Immun. *121:* 872–879 (1978).

13 Imanishi, J.; Yokota, Y.; Kishida, T.; Mukainaka, T.; Matsuo, A.: Phagocytosis-enhancing effect of human leukocyte interferon preparation of human peripheral monocytes in vitro. Acta virol., Prague *19:* 52–58 (1975).

14 Johnson, H. M.; Smith, B. G.; Baron, S.: Inhibition of the primary in vitro antibody response by interferon preparations. J. Immun. *114:* 403–409 (1975).

15 Masucci, M. G.; Masucci, G.; Klein, E.; Berthold, W.: Target selectivity of interferon-induced human killer lymphocyte related to their Fc-receptor expression. Proc. natn. Acad. Sci. USA *77:* 3620–3624 (1980).

16 Masucci, M. G.; Masucci, G.; Klein, E.; Berthold, W.: Interferon-induced cytotoxicity of human lymphocytes. In: Serou, Rosenfeld (eds.), International Symposium on New Trends in Human Immunology and Cancer Immunotherapy, pp. 887–900 (Dom Editeurs, Paris 1980).

17 McCoy, J. L.; Dean, J. H.; Herberman, R.: Human cell-mediated immunity to tuberculin as assayed by the agarose microdroplet leukocyte migration inhibition technique: Comparison with the capillary tube assay. J. immunol. Methods *15:* 335–371 (1977).

18 Nagata, S.; Taira, H.; Hall, A.; Johnsard, L.; Streuli, M.; Ecsödi, J.; Boll, W.; Cantell, K.; Weissman, Ch.: Synthesis in E. coli of a polypeptide with human leukocyte interferon activity. Nature *284:*316–320 (1980).
19 Nisbet, N. W.; Simonsen, M.; Zaleski, M.: The frequency of antigen-sensitive cells in transplantation. J. exp. Med. *129:*459–463 (1969).
20 Saksela, E.; Timonen, T.; Cantell, K.: Human natural killer-cell activity is augmented by interferon via recruitment of pre-NK cells. Scand. J. Immunol. *10:* 257–266 (1979).
21 Symington, F. W.; Teh, H. S.: A two-signal mechanism for the induction of cytotoxic T-lymphocytes. Scand. J. Immunol. *12:*1–14 (1980).
22 Søborg, M.; Bendixen, G.: Human lymphocyte migration as a parameter of hypersensitivity. Acta med. scand. *181:*247–256 (1967).
23 Targan, S.; Dorey, F.: Interferon activation of "pre-spontaneous killer" (PRE-SK) cells and alteration in kinetics of lysis of both "PRE-SK" and active cells. J. Immun. *124:*2157–2216 (1980).
24 Trinchieri, G.; Santoli, D.: Antiviral activity induced by culturing lymphocytes with tumor-derived and virus-transformed cells: Enhancement of human natural-killer-cell activity by interferon and antagonistic inhibition of susceptibility of target cells to lysis. J. exp. med. *147:*1314–1333 (1978).
25 Trinchieri, G.; Santoli, D.; Dee, R. R.; Knowles, B. B.: Antiviral activity induced by culturing lymphocytes with tumor-derived or virus-transformed cells: Identification of the antiviral activity as interferon and characterization of the human effector lymphocyte subpopulation. J. exp. med. *147:*1299–1313 (1978).
26 Vanky, F.; Argov, S.; Einhorn, S.; Klein, E.: Role of alloantigens in natural killing. Allogeneic but not autologous tumor biopsy cells are sensitive for interferon-induced cytotoxicity of human blood lymphocytes. J. exp. med. *151:* 1151–1165 (1980).
27 Vanky, F.; Klein, E.; Stjernswärd, J.; Nilsonne, U.; Rodrigez, L.; Peterffy, A.: Human tumor-lymphocyte interaction in vitro. II. Conditions which improve the capacity of biopsy cells to stimulate autologous lymphocytes. Cancer Immunol. Immunother. *5:*63–69 (1978).
28 Zarling, J. M.; Eskra, L.; Borden, E. C.; Horoszewicz, J.; Carter, W. A.: Activation of human natural killer cells cytotoxic for human leukemia cells by purified interferon. J. Immun. *123:*63–70 (1979).

Dr. Maria-Grazia Masucci, Institute for Tumor Biology, Karolinska Institute, S-10401 Stockholm

Interferons: Preclinical Rationale for Trials in Human Bladder Carcinoma

Ernest C. Borden, Norio Yamamoto, Thomas F. Hogan, Bruce S. Edwards, George T. Bryan

Division of Clinical Oncology, Department of Human Oncology, University of Wisconsin Clinical Sciences Center, and
William S. Middleton Memorial Veterans Hospital, Madison, Wisconsin, USA

Introduction

Interferons are effective inhibitors of both viral- and nonviral-induced animal tumors [10, 13]. Daily injection of mouse interferon resulted in a 33% increase in the mean survival time of L1210 leukemia-inoculated mice [11]. Survival of mice inoculated with Ehrlich-ascites tumor increased from 16 to 118 days [11]. Both the incidence of pulmonary metastases and the size of established Lewrs-lung primaries were decreased after 14 days of interferon treatment [12]. Polyribonucleotides, such as poly I: poly C, poly A: poly U, and poly ICLC are potent interferon inducers and have proven effective against a broad range of experimental tumors of spontaneous, carcinogen, and viral origin [23]. For example, treatment of mice with reticulum-cell sarcoma or L1210 leukemia with poly I: poly C esulted in prolonged survival [23, 33]. Treatment of B16 melanoma of mice with poly I: poly C resulted in a reduction in tumor size 14 days after tumor inoculation and long-term survival of some mice [2, 21]. Poly A: poly U has antitumor effects against MCDV12 leukemia, spontaneous mammary carcinoma, and transplantable melanomas [22, 30].

Because of its propensity for development of multifocal primaries, local recurrences, loco-regional invasion, and distant dissemination, bladder carcinoma remains a significant clinical problem. Progress in evaluation of new therapeutic modalities and approaches has been slow. Few studies aimed at eradication of disease in early stages have been conducted.

To evaluate more definitively the potential applicability of interferons and interferon inducers for prevention and treatment of human bladder carcinomas, we have initiated a series of experimental studies. Our initial objectives in vitro have been to define the antiproliferative effects of interferon and interferon inducers for cells of urinary tract origin and to determine susceptibility of allogeneic targets to NK- and K-cell killing of such targets by interferons and interferon inducers. In vivo we have evaluated the activity of poly I: poly C against a transplantable bladder carcinoma of mice and, in one instance, have had an opportunity to assess the effects of human leukocyte interferon against breast carcinoma recurrent in bladder wall.

Methods

Materials

Human transitional-cell carcinomas RT112 [25] and T24 [4] were grown in monolayer cultures in minimal essential media (MEM) with Earle's salts and 10% heat-inactivated fetal calf serum (FCS) supplemented with bicarbonate and gentamicin. Interferon-α (specific activity 10^6 units/mg protein) was obtained from Dr. Kari Cantell, State Serum Institute, Helsinki [5]. Interferon-β (specific activity 10^7 units/mg protein) was obtained from Drs. Julius Horoszewicz and Susan Leong, Roswell Park Memorial Institute, Buffalo [19].

Antiproliferative Effects

Confluent cells were trypsinized from 75-cm^2 flasks and seeded into 16-mm wells in 96-well trays on day 0. On day 1 (with wells approximately 50% confluent) medium was removed from each well and replaced with 0.5 ml of medium containing interferon diluted to test concentrations in MEM with 2% FCS. Triplicate cell counts were performed on triplicate wells at 72 h and 120 h after interferons were added. Cell counts were performed in a Coulter Counter Model B (Hialeah, Florida) after removal of medium from each well, washing of cells with Hanks' balanced salt solution, and trypsinization. Mean cell number for each treatment group was calculated and compared to mean cell number per well for the untreated controls. Cell viability was assessed y trypan blue exclusion.

NK- and K-Cell Assays

Human peripheral blood lymphocytes (PBL) were purified by centrifugation (700xg, 30 min, 24°C) through Ficoll-hypaque. Mononuclear cells, substantially free of contaminating granulocytes and red cells, were collected at the Ficoll-buffer interface, washed three times in PBS, and suspended in RPMI medium 1640 containing 2% FCS. NK by PBL was measured in a 6 h-chromium-release assay in which T24 transitional-carcinoma cells were used as a target. T24 cells were labeled by incubating 5×10^6 cells in 1 ml of medium with 200 micro CI/ml Na_2 ^{51}Cr for 90 min. Labeled cells were resuspended in medium, underlayed with 2 ml FCS, centrifuged at 400xg, 7 min, 24° to remove unincorporated isotope. After two such washes, target cells were diluted and added to microtiter wells at 2×10^3 cells per well for measurement of specific cytotoxicity. PBL were added to quadruplicate wells at final effector to target-cell concentrations of 100/1, 50/1, 25/1, and 12.5/1. After 6 h incubation at 37° in 5% CO_2, humidified incubator, well supernatants were collected, and supernatant ^{51}Cr release measured. Antibody-dependent cell-mediated cytotoxicity (ADCC) assays were performed similarly using a specific T24 antisera, kindly provided by *Dr. Michael Droller* [6]. Spontaneous and maximum chromium release was estimated by incubating targets alone in medium or in a solution of 5% cetrimide, respectively. Percent cytotoxicity due to PBL is calculated according to the following formula:

$$\% \text{ cytotoxicity} = \frac{\text{test well CPM} - \text{spontaneous CPM}}{\text{maximum CPM} - \text{spontaneous CPM} \times 100}$$

Spontaneous CPM was usually less than 10 to 20% of maximum CPM.

Animal-Tumor Assays

MBT-2 transplantable mouse bladder carcinoma was kindly provided by Mark S. Soloway. Tumor-cell suspensions for inoculation were prepared by finely mincing aseptically excised tumor tissue with scissors, trypsinizing in Hanks' balanced salt solution (HBSS) containing 0.1% trypsin-EDTA and filtering through fine mesh after 20 min. A second trypsinization was performed, following which the cells were washed twice in HBSS, and the number of viable cells quantitated in a hemocytometer with viability determined by trypan blue exclusion. No preparation with less than 85% cell viability was used. Final cell concentration was adjusted to 10^5 viable cells per 0.1 cc, and 0.1 cc was inoculated subcutaneously on the backs of 20- to 22-g female C 3H/He/J mice [28]. Groups of 20 mice were then treated on alternate days with poly I: poly C (10 mg/kg).

Results

Antiproliferative Effects

RT112 cells were treated with interferon-α at 0, 10, 100, or 1000 units/ml or interferon-β at 0, 1, 10, and 100 units/ml. Both interferons inhibited proliferation of these cells (fig. 1). At all concentrations and at both time points, interferon-β had significantly greater antiproliferative activity than interferon-α. At 50% inhibition of cell growth, interferon-β was approximately 10-fold more effective than an equivalent concentration of interferon-α. These cell-count observations were confirmed by microscopic monitoring of cultures. In each instance the cell viability in all wells was unaffected by interferons and was greater than 95%.

NK- and K-Cell Augmentation

Poly I: poly C, a potent interferon inducer, augmented both the NK- and K-cell response to T24 bladder carcinoma cells. At an optimal poly I: poly C concentration (100 μg/ml), cytotoxicity increased linearly with effector: target cell ratio in a representative experiment (fig. 2). Baseline NK-cell responses were consistently low. The observed range, 0 to 10% cytotoxicity, was similar to baseline NK-cell responses typically obtained with other human tumor cell lines of non-hematologic origin (e. g. Chang hepatoma cells, A549 bronchogenic carcinoma cells, RDMS rhabdomyosarcoma cells). In 7 in-

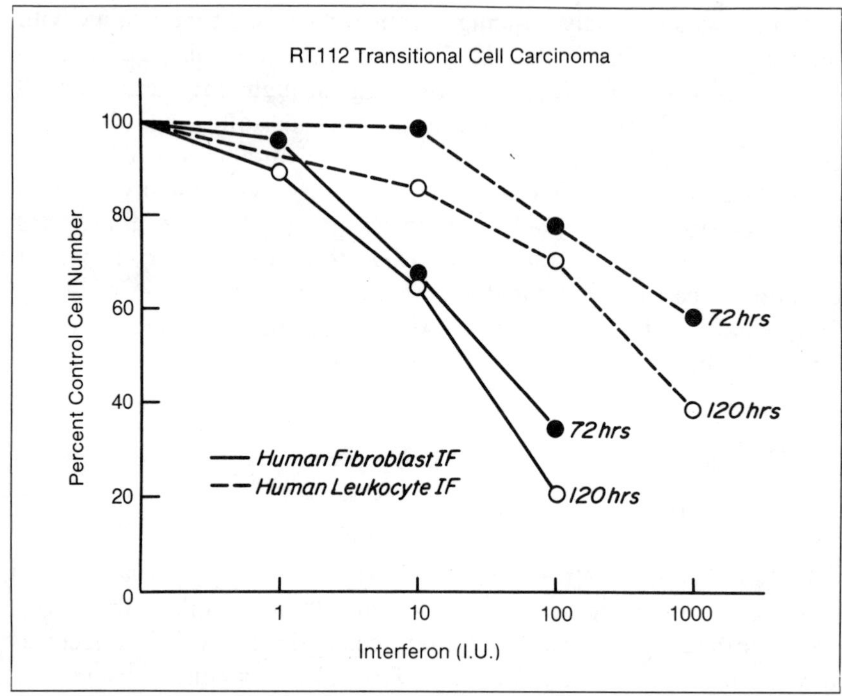

Figure 1. Antiproliferative effects of human interferon-α (- - -) and -β (—) for human RT112 transitional-carcinoma cells. Cell counts performed 72 h (●) and 120 h (○) after interferons.

Figure 2. Effect of poly I: poly C on NK- and K-cell cytotoxic responses to T24, a human bladder carcinoma cell line. Peripheral mononuclear cells from a healthy male donor were Ficoll-hypaque-purified and enriched for the presence of NK- and K-cells by centrifugation over a Percoll buoyant-density step gradient. Cells with specific densities less than 1.069 g/cm^3 were incubated 18 h with (●) or without (○) 100 μg/ml poly I: poly C, washed, and assessed for spontaneous (SCC) and antibody-dependent (ADCC) cellular cytotoxicity in parallel 6 h-^{51}Cr-release assays. Results for ADCC are illustrated both before (solid line) and after (dashed lines) mathematically correcting for parallel SCC. Corrected % ADCC = [(%ADCC − %SCC)/(100 − %SCC)]x100.

Figure 3. Antitumor effects of poly I: poly C for MBT-2 mouse bladder carcinoma. Serial tumor measurements performed after injection of 10^5 cells subcutaneously on day 1. Poly I: poly C (10 mg/kg) administered intraperitoneally on days 1, 3, and 5 (□) or days 1, 3, 5, 7, 9, 11, 13, 15, and 17 (Δ) and compared to phosphate-buffered saline-treated controls (o). Tumor measurements are means derived from 20 animals/treatment group.

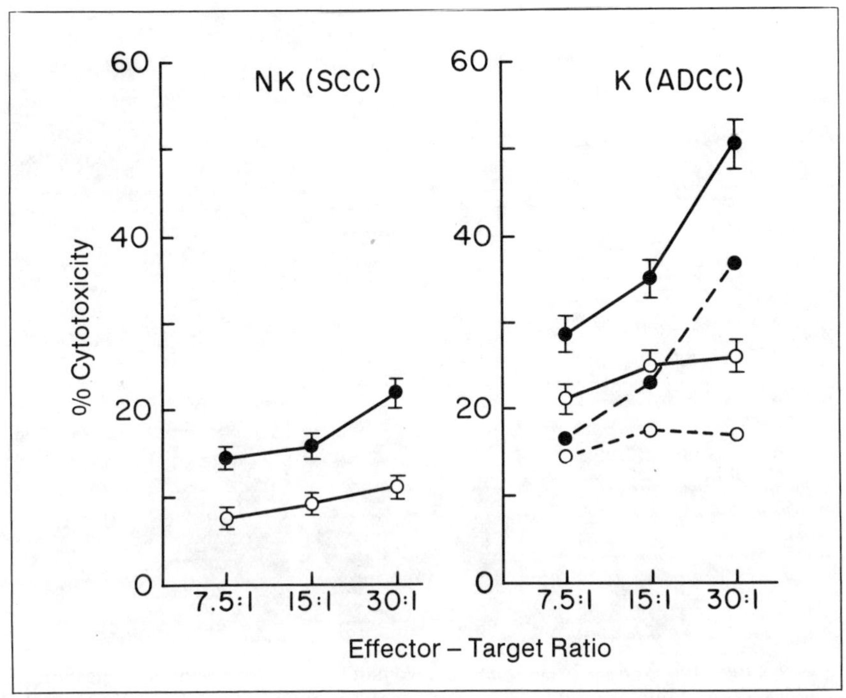
60
NK (SCC)
40
% Cytotoxicity
20
0
7.5:1
15:1
30:1
60
K (ADCC)
40
20
0
7.5:1
15:1
30:1
Effector – Target Ratio

2

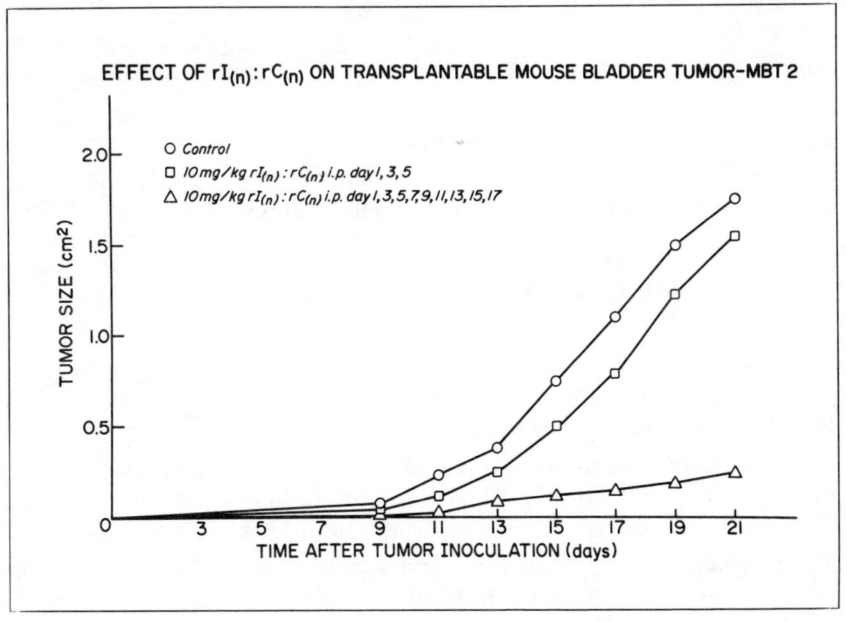
EFFECT OF $rI_{(n)}:rC_{(n)}$ ON TRANSPLANTABLE MOUSE BLADDER TUMOR-MBT 2
○ Control
□ 10 mg/kg $rI_{(n)}:rC_{(n)}$ i.p. day 1, 3, 5
△ 10 mg/kg $rI_{(n)}:rC_{(n)}$ i.p. day 1, 3, 5, 7, 9, 11, 13, 15, 17
TUMOR SIZE (cm^2)
2.0
1.5
1.0
0.5
0
3
5
7
9
11
13
15
17
19
21
TIME AFTER TUMOR INOCULATION (days)

3

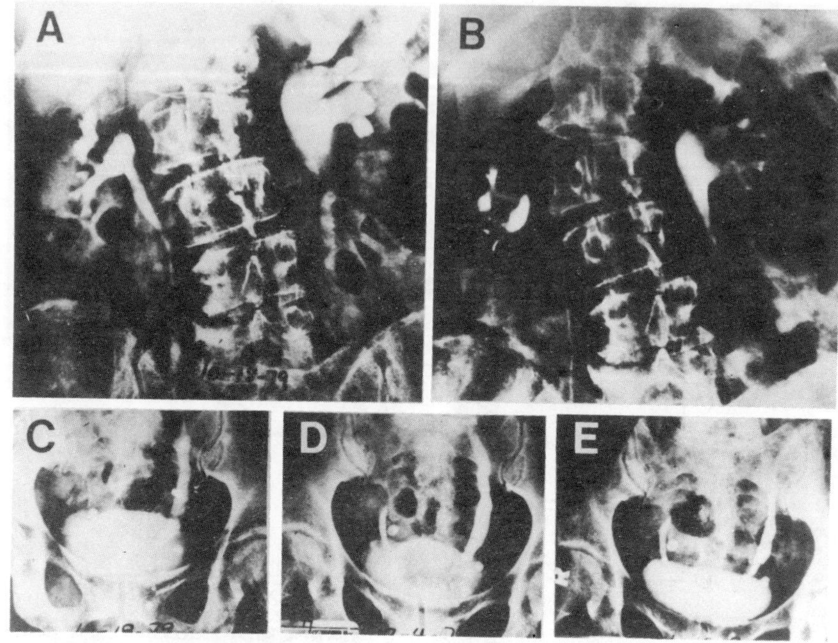

Figure 4. Intravenous pyelograms in a woman with breast carcinoma metastatic to bladder. Prior to interferon-α (A, C). After 6 weeks of interferon-α (D). After 10 weeks of interferon-α (B, E).

dividuals tested for T24-cell reactivity, NK-cell responses of 6 (86%) and K-cell responses of 2 (29%) were significantly augmented as a result of in vitro incubation of effector cells with poly I: poly C.

Antitumor Effects in Vivo

Intraperitoneal administration of poly I: poly C (10 mg/kg) began 24 h after subcutaneous implantation of 10^5 MBT-2 tumor cells. Poly I: poly C was given for a total of 3 or 9 injections on alternate days. Repeated injections for 17 days resulted in significant inhibition of MBT-2 growth (fig. 3). A more limited period of injection resulted in no effect. Similar results were obtained when 10^4 tumor cells were implanted. Repeated experiments with both 10^4 and 10^5 tumor cells resulted in identical findings.

One patient in the American Cancer Society trial of interferon-α for metastatic breast carcinoma had an unusual site of secondary involvement. Cystoscopy, performed because of symptoms of frequency and urgency, revealed mucosal involvement of carcinoma which on biopsy proved to be consistent with her original breast carcinoma primary. Intravenous pyelogram demonstrated bilateral hydronephrosis. Interferon administration resulted in marked improvement in her symptoms of urgency, frequency, and nocturia. This was accompanied by objective improvement in her hydroureter and hydronephrosis (fig. 4). These observations suggest that bladder-wall involvement by carcinoma can be influenced by systemic administration of interferons.

Discussion

Elucidating the roles of interferons and interferon inducers in treatment of bladder carcinomas could be enhanced by the well-studied experimental models of etiology and pathogenesis [3]. Use of suitable animal models has contributed to recent rapid advances in the successful chemotherapy of human malignancies. Drugs active in animal models have proven effective in clinical trials [8].

Two major cellular mechanisms of antitumor action of interferons have been identified: direct antiproliferative effects and immunomodulatory effects. Interferons clearly have antiproliferative effects for in vitro cell replication [1, 7, 17, 29]. The antiproliferative effects track with the antiviral effects during purification of naturally produced interferons. Enhancement after interferon treatment of cell destruction by human immune effector cells has been widely demonstrated in vitro and, to a more limited extent, in vivo. Cytotoxic function of T-cells, NK-cells, K-cells, and macrophages has been augmented by interferons [14, 15, 27, 31, 32]. Interferons and interferon inducers seem to play a pivotal role in regulating the maturation and activity of NK-cells.

To achieve tumor regression in vivo, the relative importance of inhibition of cell proliferation, when compared to immunoaugmentation, requires further evaluation. Interferons themselves inhibited proliferation of bladder carcinoma cells. Whether NK- and K-cells or other immune effector cell subpopulations are also important will require further assessment. Since fresh bladder-carcinoma cells are easily obtainable at surgery, by barbotage, and by cystoscopy, human bladder carcinoma offers an unusual opportunity not only to dissect the relative role of the immunoaugmenting and antiproliferative effects of interferon and interferon inducers, but also to evaluate the effects of various immune effector cell subpopulations for fresh tumor-cell targets.

Differences in antiproliferative effects of interferons-α and -β for lymphoblastoid and osteosarcoma cells have been reported [7]. Greater antiproliferative effects of interferon-β for carcinoma cells of urinary-tract origin suggest that interferon-β may have greater antiproliferative effects than naturally produced interferon-α for a wider variety of malignant cells. Whether interferon-α subspecies, obtained by recombinant DNA techniques, will prove to have greater growth inhibitory effects than interferon-β will require additional evaluation.

Corroborative observations support the possibility of successful application of interferons and interferon inducers for treatment of bladder carcinoma. Human interferon-β inhibited growth of two human transitional carcinomas in nude mice [18]. Intravesical administration of poly I: poly C and of human interferon-α resulted in possible reduction in frequency of recurrences of bladder papillomas following initial fulguration [20, 24]. A patient with bladder carcinoma, treated with interferon-α with objective tumor regression, has been reported [16].

Little work has been performed to determine the effects of interferons and interferon inducers in inhibiting chemical oncogenesis. Induction of fibrosarcomas and pulmonary adenomas in CF-1 mice by 3-methylcholanthrene was inhibited by interferon treatment [26]. None of the treated mice developed tumors, whereas 17 of 18 controls did [26]. Poly I: poly C, given for a limited period after dimethylbenzanthracene, inhibited tumorigenesis in Swiss mice [9]. Rat and mouse bladder carcinomas can be reproducibly induced by chemical carcinogens [3]. Experimental models should help dissect the possible role of interferons and interferon inducers as chemoprophylactic agents in bladder carcinoma.

Acknowledgments

Research activities supported by NIH grants CA 14520, CA 14524, CA 20432, the Medical Research Service of the Veterans Administration, and the American Cancer Society. Technical assistance, essential for completion of these experiments, was provided by *Kimberly Sack* and *Edward Grunden*. We are grateful to *Dr. E. Ertürk* for histologic examination of MBT-2 tumors. The manuscript was ably prepared by *Mary Ann Liposcak*.

References

1 Balkwill, F. R.; Oliver, R. T. D.: Growth-inhibitory effects of interferon on normal and malignant human haemopoietic cells. Int. J. Cancer *20:*500–505 (1977).

2 Bart, R. S.; Kopf, A. W.; Vilcek, J. T.; Lam, S.: Role of interferon in the antimelanoma effects of poly (I): poly (C) and Newcastle disease virus. Nature new Biol. *245:*229–230 (1973).

3 Bryan, G. T.: The pathogenesis of experimental bladder cancer. Cancer Res. *37:* 2813–2816 (1977).

4 Bubenik, J.; Baresova, M.; Viklicky, V.; Jakoubkova, J.; Sainerova, H.; Donner, J.: Established cell line of urinary bladder carcinoma (T24) containing tumour-specific antigen. Int. J. Cancer *11:*765–773 (1973).

5 Cantell, K.; Hirvonen S.; Morensen, K. E.; Phyälä, L.: Human leukocyte interferon: Production, purification, stability, and animal experiments in the production and use of interferon for the treatment and prevention of human virus infections. In: Waymouth (ed.), Proceedings of a Tissue Culture Association Workshop *3:*35–38 (1973).

6 Droller, M. J.; Borg, H.; Perlmann, P.: In vitro enhancement of natural and antibody-dependent lymphocyte-mediated cytotoxicity against tumor target cells by interferon. Cell. Immunol. *47:*248–260 (1979).

7 Einhorn, S.; Strander, H.: Is interferon tissue specific? Effect of human leukocyte and fibroblast interferons on the growth of lymphoblastoid and osteosarcoma cell lines. J. gen. Virol. *34:*573–577 (1977).

8 Frei, E., III; Schabel, F. M., Jr.; Goldin A.: Comparative chemotherapy of AKR lymphoma and human hematological neoplasia. Cancer Res. *34:*184–193 (1974).

9 Gelboin, H. V.; Levy, H. B.: Polyinosinic-polycytidylic acid inhibits chemically induced tumorigenesis in mouse skin. Science *167:*205–207 (1970).

10 Gresser, I.: Antitumor effects of interferon. Adv. Cancer Res. *16:*97–140 (1972).

11 Gresser, I.; Bourali, C.: Antitumor effects of interferon preparations in mice. J. natn. Cancer Inst. *45:*365–376 (1970).

12 Gresser, I.; Bourali-Maury, C.: Inhibition by interferon preparations of a solid malignant tumour and pulmonary metastases in mice. Nature, Lond. *236:*78–79 (1972).

13 Gresser, I.; Tovey, M. G.: Antitumor effects of interferon. Biochem. biophys. Acta *516:*231–247 (1978).

14 Herberman, R. B.; Ortaldo, J. R.; Bonnard, G. D.: Augmentation by interferon of human natural and antibody-dependent cell-mediated cytotoxicity. Nature *277:* 221–223 (1979).

15 Herberman, R. B.; Ortaldo, J. R.; Djeu, J. Y.; Holden, H. T.; Jett, J.; Lang, N. P.; Rubinstein, M.; Pestka, S.: Role of interferon in regulation of natural-killer cells and macrophages. Ann. N. Y. Acad. Sci. *350:*63–71 (1980).

16 Hill, N. O.; Pardue, A.; Khan, A.; Aleman, C.; Dorn, G.; Hill, J. M.: Phase-I human leukocyte interferon trials in cancer and leukemia. J. clin. Hemat. Oncol. *11:*23–35 (1981).

17 Horoszewicz, J. S.; Leong, S. S.; Carter, W. A.: Noncycling tumor cells are sensitive targets for the antiproliferative activity of human interferon. Science *206:* 1091–1093 (1979).

18 Horoszewicz, J.; Leong, S. S.; Ito, M.; Buffett, R. F.; Karakousis, C.; Holyoke, E.; Job, L.; Dolen, J. G.; Carter, W. A.: Human fibroblast interferon in human neoplasia: Clinical and laboratory study. Cancer Treatm. Rep. *62:* 1899–1906 (1978).

19 Horoszewicz, J.; Leong, S. S.; Ito, M.; Diberardino, L.; Carter, W. A.: Aging in vitro and large-scale interferon production by 15 new strains of human diploid fibroblasts. Infect. Immunity *19:* 720–726 (1978).

20 Kemeny, N.; Yagoda, A.; Whitmore, W.; Grabstald, H.; Young, C.; Krakoff, I.: Randomized prospective therapeutic trial of poly rI: rC in patients with papillomas or superficial carcinomas of the urinary bladder. Proc. Amer. Ass. Cancer Res. *17:* 171 (1976).

21 Kreider, J. W.; Benjamin, S. A.: Tumor immunity and the mechanism of polyinosinic-polycytidylic acid inhibition of tumor growth. J. natn. Cancer Inst. *49:* 1303–1310 (1972).

22 Lacour, F.; Spira, A.; Lacour, J.; Prade, M.: Polyadenylic-polyuridylic acid, an adjunct to surgery in the treatment of spontaneous mammary tumors in C3H/He mice and transplantable melanoma in the hamster. Cancer Res. *32:* 648–649 (1972).

23 Levy, H. B.; Asofsky, R.; Riley, F.; Garapin, A.; Canto, H.; Adamson, R.: The mechanism of the antitumor action of poly I: poly C. Ann. N. Y. Acad. Sci. *172:* 640–648 (1970).

24 Nola, P.; Ikie, D.; Kensevic, M.; Maricic, Z.; Jusic, D.; Soos, E.: Therapy of papillomatosis of the urinary bladder with human leukocyte interferon. Personal communication, Interferon Scientific Memoranda (June, 1978).

25 Rigby, C. C.; Franks, L. M.: A human tissue culture cell line from a transitional cell tumour of the urinary bladder: Growth, chromosome pattern, and ultrastructure. Br. J. Cancer *24:* 746–754 (1970).

26 Salerno, R. A.; Whitmire, C. E.; Garcia, I. M.; Huebner, R. J.: Chemical carcinogenesis in mice inhibited by interferon. Nature new Biol. *239:* 31–32 (1972).

27 Schultz, R. M.; Pavlidis, N. A.; Stylos, W. A.; Chirigos, M. A.: Regulation of macrophage tumoricidal function: A role for prostaglandins of the E series. Science *202:* 320–321 (1978).

28 Soloway, M. S.: Intravesical and systemic chemotherapy of murine bladder cancer. Cancer Res. *37:* 2918–2929 (1977).

29 Strander, H.; Einhorn, S.: Effect of human leukocyte interferon on the growth of human osteosarcoma cells in tissue culture. Int. J. Cancer *19:* 468–473 (1977).

30 Webb, D.; Braun, W.; Plescia, O. J.: Antitumor effects of polynucleotides and theophylline. Cancer Res. *32:* 1814–1819 (1972).

31 Zarling, J. M.; Eskra, L.; Borden, E. C.; Horoszewicz, J.; Carter, W. A.: Activation of human natural-killer cells cytotoxic for human leukemia cells by purified interferon. J. Immun. *123:* 63–70 (1979).

32 Zarling, J. M.; Sosman, J.; Eskra, L.; Borden, E. C.; Horoszewicz, J. S.; Carter, W. A.: Enhancement of T-cell cytotoxic responses by purified human fibroblast interferon. J. Immun. *121:* 2002–2004 (1978).

33 Zeleznick, L. D.; Bhuyan, B. K.: Treatment of leukemic (L1210) mice with double-stranded polyribonucleotides. Proc. Soc. exp. Biol. Med. *130:* 126–128 (1969).

Prof. Dr. Ernest C. Borden, Division of Clinical Oncology, Department of Human Oncology, University of Wisconsin Clinical Sciences Center, USA- Madison, Wisconsin 53792

Interferon Potentiation: Antiviral and Antitumor Studies[1]

W. R. Fleischmann, Jr.

Department of Microbiology, University of Texas Medical Branch, Galveston, Texas, USA

Introduction

The antiviral properties of interferons were discovered by *Isaacs* and *Lindenmann* in 1957 [18]. Interferons have also been shown to have potent immunoregulatory properties and antitumor activities [for reviews see 3, 14, 19]. More than twenty years of research effort have added much to the understanding of interferons and their actions, however, the precise mechanisms by which interferons exert their actions are still largely unknown.

Interferons are natural substances produced by virtually all cells of a wide range of vertebrates. Three types of interferons have been identified [29]: leukocyte interferon (IFN-α), fibroblast interferon (IFN-β), and immune interferon (IFN-γ). Leukocyte and fibroblast interferons are also called virus-type interferons because they can be induced by viruses and polyribonucleotides [2, 6–8, 12, 15–18, 22, 24–26, 31]. In man, leukocyte and fibroblast interferons are produced by leukocytes and by fibroepithelial cells, respectively. In the mouse, leukocyte and fibroblast interferons are produced as a mixture in virus-induced interferon preparations [21]. Immune interferon is induced in both man and mouse by exposing lymphocytes to T-cell mitogens such as staphylococcal enterotoxin A, phytohemagglutin P, and concanavalin A or to specific antigens to which the lymphocytes have been sensitized [13, 20, 27, 30, 33].

[1] Supported by NIH Grant 5S07 RR-05427 and CA-26475 and by American Cancer Society Grant IN 112B.

This paper describes a novel interaction of virus-type and immune interferons which, when used in combination, caused a synergistic enhancement or potentiation of the antiviral and antitumor activities of the interferons. Potentiation has been well documented for the mouse interferon system. Potentiation factors ranged from 5- to greater than 20-fold depending on the concentrations of the interferons employed. Further, preliminary studies with the human system have given analogous results.

Potentiation of Antiviral Activity of Interferon

Potentiation was first demonstrated as a non-additive synergistic enhancement of the antiviral activity of mixed preparations of mouse virus-type and immune interferons [9]. Mouse L-cells were treated with growth medium, immune interferon alone, virus-type interferon alone, or a combination of immune and virus type interferon. The immune interferon had been prepared by stimulating mouse spleen cells with staphylococcal enterotoxin A. The virus-type interferon had

Table I. Potentiation of interferon activity by mixed preparations of immune interferon and virus-type interferon[a]

IF sample	Virus yield (PFU/ml)	Fold inhibition	IF titer (U/ml)		Fold potentiation[d]
			Actual[b]	Expected[c]	
No IF	$1.0 \times 10^9 \pm 0.1 \times 10^9$[e]	–	–	–	–
Immune IF	$3.8 \times 10^8 \pm 0.4 \times 10^8$	2.6	3	–	–
Virus-type IF	$2.3 \times 10^7 \pm 0.1 \times 10^7$	43	26	–	–
Immune IF + virus-type IF	$1.4 \times 10^6 \pm 0.03 \times 10^6$	714	320	29	11

[a] Mouse L-cell monolayers were treated for 12 h with growth medium (no interferon [IF]), immune interferon, virus-type interferon, and immune interferon and virus-type interferon in combination. The monolayers were challenged with mengovirus at a multiplicity of infection 10 PFU/cell, and virus yields were harvested 24 h later.

[b] Actual interferon titers were determined by comparison of virus yield with a standard yield reduction curve of interferon activity determined concurrently.

[c] Expected interferon titer was determined by adding the actual titers of the interferon present in the mixed interferon preparation.

[d] The potentiation factor was determined by dividing the actual interferon titer by the expected interferon titer.

[e] Mean ± standard deviation [with permission from ref. 9].

been prepared by challenging L-cells with Newcastle disease virus. As shown in table I, 3 units of immune interferon provided a 2.6-fold inhibition of mengovirus yield and 25 units of virus-type interferon provided a 43-fold inhibition. The combination of immune and virus-type interferons would have been expected, on the basis of the additivity of the two interferons, to provide 29 units of protective effect. Therefore, an approximately 50-fold inhibition was expected. Instead, an approximately 700-fold inhibition was observed. This level of inhibition corresponded to the protective effect of 320 units of either immune or virus-type interferon alone. Thus, the immune and virus-type interferons employed in combination caused an 11-fold greater than expected protective effect.

A number of interpretations of the potentiation phenomenon were possible. Previous reports had described the potentiating effect on interferon of cyclic AMP [1, 11, 23, 32] and of antimetabolites such as actinomycin D [5]. Further, many lymphokines which might have potentiating activity were present with immune interferon in the mitogen-stimulated mouse spleen cell supernatant fluids. It was important to determine whether potentiation was a function of the interferons themselves or of a substance(s) separable from the interferons.

Table II. Effect of partial purification of virus-type interferon on potentiation[a]

IF sample	Virus yield (PFU/ml)	Fold inhibition	IF titer (U/ml)		Fold potentiation
			Actual	Expected	
No IF	$7.7 \times 10^8 \pm 0.3 \times 10^8$[b]	–	–	–	–
Immune IF	$1.6 \times 10^8 \pm 0.2 \times 10^8$	4.8	9	–	–
Purified virus-type IF	$5.5 \times 10^7 \pm 0.2 \times 10^7$	14	17	–	–
Virus-type IF	$5.9 \times 10^7 \pm 0.3 \times 10^7$	13	16	–	–
Immune IF + purified virus-type IF	$2.1 \times 10^6 \pm 0.2 \times 10^6$	370	130	26	5
Immune IF + virus-type IF	$2.2 \times 10^6 \pm 0.7 \times 10^6$	345	130	25	5

[a] Mouse L-cell monolayers were treated for 12 h with growth medium (no interferon [IF]), immune interferon, 10,000-fold purified virus-type interferon, unpurified virus-type interferon, immune interferon plus purified virus-type interferon in combination, and immune interferon and unpurified virus-type interferon in combination. The monolayers were challenged with mengovirus at a multiplicity of infection of 10 PFU/cell, and virus yields were harvested 24 h later.

[b] Mean ± standard deviation [with permission from ref. 9].

To address this question, partially purified virus-type interferon (specific activity = 10^7 U/mg of protein) and crude virus-type interferon were employed in a potentiation experiment. As shown in table II, identical levels of potentiation were observed when each of the virus-type interferon preparations were combined with crude immune interferon. Since the virus-type interferon had been purified 10,000-fold with no loss of potentiating ability, it was unlikely that the potentiation phenomenon was the result of a factor separable from virus-type interferon.

Next, the immune interferon preparation was evaluated for the identity of the potentiation factor as either interferon or a substance separable from interferon. This was addressed in two ways. The first dealt with the relative stabilities of the potentiation factor and immune interferon under a variety of conditions. Both activities demonstrated stability at 50°C, identical kinetics of inactivation at 60°C, identical kinetics of inactivation at pH 2, and identical kinetics of inactivation by antibody to crude immune interferon. The second way of addressing this problem was to follow the two activities as crude immune interferon was subjected to a variety of chromatographic techniques. The potentiation factor and immune interferon were not

Table III. Effect of partial purification of immune interferon on potentiation[a]

IF sample	Virus yield (PFU/ml)	Fold inhibition	IF titer (U/ml)		Fold-potentiation
			Actual	Expected	
No IF	$6.8 \times 10^8 \pm 0.00$[b]	–	–	–	–
Immune IF	$3.6 \times 10^8 \pm 0.2 \times 10^8$	1.8	6	–	–
Purified immune IF	$3.9 \times 10^8 \pm 0.2 \times 10^8$	1.8	5	–	–
Virus-type IF	$4.9 \times 10^7 \pm 1.5 \times 10^7$	14	20	–	–
Immune IF + virus-type IF	$1.3 \times 10^6 \pm 0.05 \times 10^6$	526	480	26	18
Purified immune IF + virus-type IF	$1.4 \times 10^6 \pm 0.04 \times 10^6$	476	450	25	18

[a] Mouse L-cell monolayers were treated for 12 h with growth medium (no interferon [IF], unpurified immune interferon, 200-fold-purified immune interferon from an Ultrogel filtration immune interferon, virus-type interferon, unpurified immune interferon plus virus-type interferon in combination, and partially purified immune interferon plus virus-type interferon in combination. The monolayers were challenged with mengovirus at a multiplicity of infection of 10 PFU/cell, and virus yields were harvested 24 h later.

[b] Mean ± standard deviation [with permission from ref. 9].

separated by chromatography on Affigel 202; DEAE-cellulose; DEAE-sephadex; and Amicon affinity chromatography Matrix Gel dyes, Red, Blue A, Blue B, Green, and Orange. Further, the purification scheme of differentiated ammonium sulfate precipitation and chromatography on Ultrogel AcA 34 gave a 200-fold purification of immune interferon, but did not affect the relative ratio of potentiation factor to interferon (table III). While these data cannot be regarded as definitive evidence that the potentiation factor is inseparable from immune interferon, they do indicate that, if the two activities reside on different molecules, the two molecules must have very similar properties.

Preliminary studies on the mode of action of potentiation suggest that potentiation is directly dependent on the concentration of each of the two types of interferon [28]. This data, taken together with the results described above, indicate that it is the synergistic interaction of the immune and virus-type interferons which is the most likely explanation of the potentiation phenomenon.

Potentiation of Antitumor Action of Interferon

It was important to determine whether the potentiation phenomenon was a general feature of the interaction of immune and virus-type interferons or if it was restricted to their antiviral activities. Each interferon, employed alone, had been shown by many others to have a marked antitumor activity [14]. Potentiation studies on the antitumor activity of interferon employed two mouse tumor systems: the first a developing tumor and the second an established tumor.

In the first mouse tumor system, DBA/2 mice were inoculated subcutaneously with 10^5 P388 leukemia cells [10]. They were treated daily at the site of tumor implantation for 16 days with mock interferon, virus-type interferon alone (25,000 units/day), immune interferon alone (25 units/day), or the combination of immune (25 units/day) and virus-type interferons (25,000 units/day). Tumors developed as a solid mass and tumor size was monitored. The day of death of the mice was also noted. As shown in fig. 1 and fig. 2, virus-type interferon provided a statistically significant antitumor effect as measured by both a 3-day delay in tumor cell growth and a 2.4-day increased survival time. The low dose of immune interferon alone pro-

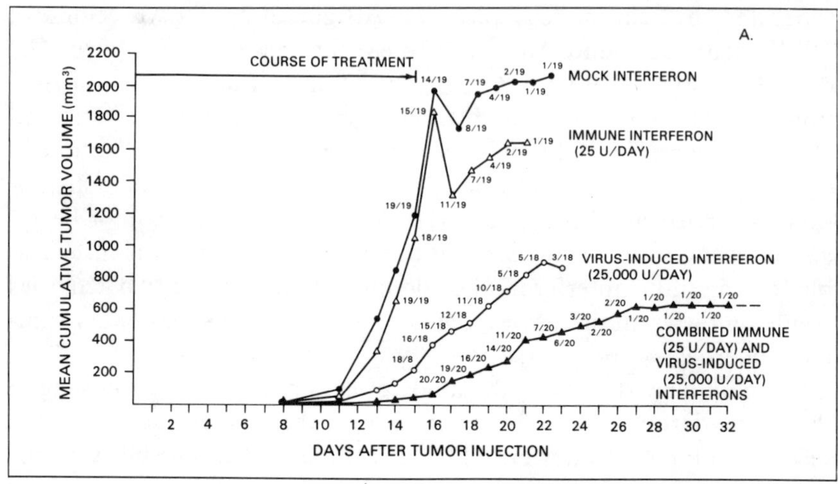

Figure 1. Effect of combined immune and virus-induced interferons on the rate of P388 tumor development in DBA/2 mice. Each mouse was inoculated sc with 10^5 P388 tumor cells, and they were then divided into 4 groups of 18 – 20 each. Mice were inoculated 3 h before tumor injection and daily for 15 days thereafter at the approximate site of tumor injection with mock interferon (●), immune interferon (△), virus-induced interferon (○), or a combination of immune and virus-induced interferons (▲). Volume of the primary tumor was determined for each mouse on the indicated days after tumor cell injection. Data were plotted as the linear increase in mean cumulative tumor volume. Mean cumulative tumor volumes were determined within each group by averaging the tumor size of all surviving mice with the final tumor size of all mice that had died. Fractions indicate no. of survivors/total no. of mice at the indicated times after tumor injection for each treatment group [10].

vided no antitumor effect. However, when the immune interferon was combined with virus-type interferon, the combination potentiated the antitumor activity. This was demonstrated by an additional 3-day delay in tumor cell growth and by an additional 2.1-day increased survival time relative to that observed for virus-type interferon alone.

In the second mouse tumor system, established squamous-cell carcinomas induced in hairless mice by irradiation with UV light were treated by intralesional injection with mock interferon, virus-type interferon (3000 units/day), immune interferon (10 units/day), or a combination of immune (10 units/day) and virus-type interferons (3000 units/day) [4]. As shown in figure 3, after 19 days of treatment, tumors injected with immune interferon alone and with mock interferon demonstrated a 20% reduction in tumor size. This slight regression might reflect an inflammatory response triggered by proteins

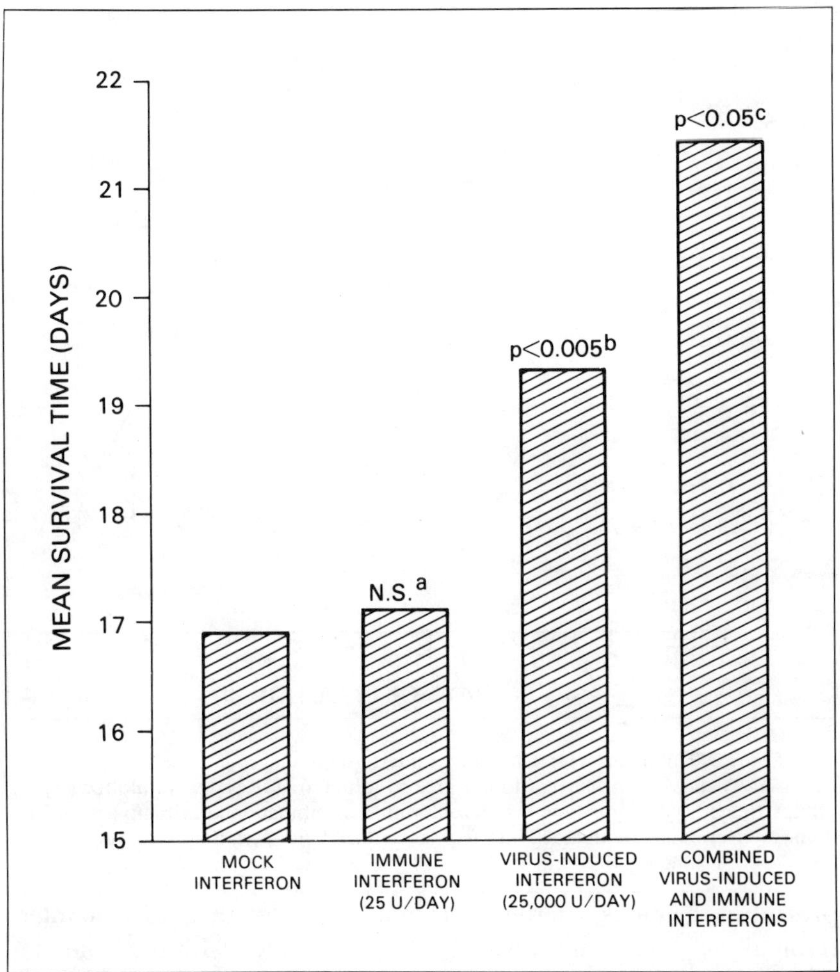

Figure 2. Effect of combined immune and virus-induced interferons on life-spans of mice inoculated with P388 tumor cells. Each mouse was inoculated sc with 10^5 P388 tumor cells, and they were then divided into 4 groups of 18 – 20 each. Mice were inoculated daily for 15 days at the approximate site of tumor injection with mock interferon, 25 U immune interferon/day, 25,000 U virus-induced interferon/day, or a combination of 25 U immune interferon/day and 25,000 U virus-induced interferon/day. Day of death of each mouse was noted. Results were plotted as the mean survival time for each of the 4 groups of mice. Statistical probabilities were determined by the t-test. Comparable statistical probabilities were observed when the data were analyzed by the Mann-Whitney U test. Immune interferon treatment was compared to mock interferon treatment (a). NS = not significant. Virus-induced interferon treatment was compared to mock interferon treatment (b). Combined-interferon treatment was compared to virus-induced interferon treatment (c) [10].

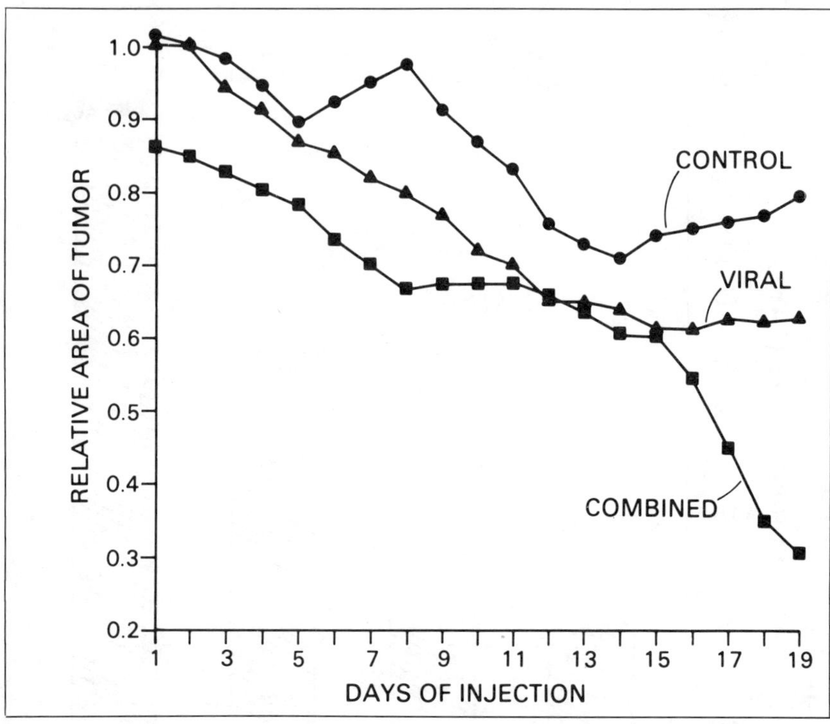

Figure 3. Tumor size regression under interferon management. Regression is characterized by the ratio of current tumor area to initial area. Results are plotted for the groups treated with virus-type interferon, with a combination of virus-type and immune interferon, and with mock interferons (control) [with permission from Ref. 4].

present in the mock interferon. Tumors treated with virus-type interferon alone were reduced by 38%. Tumors treated with the combination of immune and virus-type interferons demonstrated a potentiation of the antitumor effect as they were reduced in size by 69%, a value significantly greater than that observed for virus-type interferon alone.

Discussion

Combined preparations of immune and virus-type interferons caused a potentiation not only of the antiviral activity of the interferons but also of their antitumor activity. Potentiation of the antitumor activity of interferon was demonstrable against both developing and established mouse tumors. The mechanism of potentiation is not yet understood, however, the phenomenon has considerable potential significance. As mentioned above, preliminary work with human immune interferon suggested that potentiation also occurred with the human interferon systems. While the mouse studies must be vigorously confirmed for their application to the human system before final judgments can be made, these results hold the promise that combined interferon therapy in man might increase the efficacy of the interferon therapy against viral diseases and cancer.

References

1 Allen, L. B.; Eagle, N. C.; Huffman, J. H.; Shuman, D. A.; Meyer, R. B., Jr.; Sidwell, R. W.: Enhancement of interferon antiviral action in L-cells by cyclic nucleotides. Proc. Soc. exp. Biol. Med. *146:* 580–584 (1974).

2 Ash, R. J.; Bubel, H. C.: Temporal relationship of interferon production and resistance to experimentally induced virus infection. J. infect. Dis. *116:* 1–7 (1966).

3 Baron, S.; Dianzani, F.: General considerations of the interferon system. Tex. Rep. Biol. Med. *35:* 1–10 (1977).

4 Brysk, M. M.; Tschen, E. H.; Hudson, R. D.; Smith, E. B.; Fleischmann, W. R., Jr.; Black, H. S.: The activity of interferon on U-V light-induced squamous carcinomas in mice. J. Am. Acad. Dermat. *5:* 61–63 (1981).

5 Chany, C.; Fournier, F.; Rousset, S.: Potentiation of the antiviral activity of interferon by actinomycin D. Nature *230:* 113–114 (1971).

6 Falcoff, E.; Fournier, F.; Chany, C.: Étude comparative des poids moleculaires de deux interferons humains produits in vitro. Ann. Inst. Pasteur, Paris *111:* 241–248 (1966).

7 Field, A. K.; Lampson, G. P.; Tytell, A. A.; Nemes, M. M.; Hilleman, M. R.: Inducers of interferon and host resistance. IV. Double-stranded replicative form RNA (MS2-RF-RNA) from E. coli infected with MS2 coliphage. Proc. natn. Acad. Sci. USA *58:* 2101–2108 (1967).

8 Field, A. K.; Tytell, A. A.; Lampson, G. P.; Hilleman, M. R.: Inducers of interferon and host resistance. II. Multistranded synthetic polynucleotide complexes. Proc. natn. Acad. Sci. USA *58:* 1004–1010 (1967).

9 Fleischmann, W. R.; Jr.; Georgiades, J. A.; Osborne, L. C.; Johnson, H. M.: Potentiation of interferon activity by mixed preparations of fibroblast and immune interferon. Infect. Immunity *26:* 248–253 (1979).

10 Fleischmann, W. R.; Jr.; Kleyn, K. M.; Baron, S.: Potentiation of antitumor effect of virus-induced interferon by mouse immune interferon preparations. J. natn. Cancer Inst. *65:* 963–966 (1980).

11 Friedman, R. M.; Pastan, I.: Interferon and cyclic-3'5'-adenosine monophosphate: Potentiation of antiviral activity. Biochem. biophys. Res. Commun. *36:* 735–740 (1969).

12 Glasgow, L. A.: Leukocytes and interferon in the host response to viral infections. I. Mouse leukocytes and leukocyte-produced interferon in vaccinia virus infection in vitro. J. exp. Med. *121:* 1001–1018 (1965).

13 Green J. A.; Cooperband, S. R.; Kibrick, S.: Immune-specific induction of interferon production in cultures of human blood lymphocytes. Science *164:* 1415 – 1417 (1969).

14 Gresser, I.; Tovey, M. G.: Antitumor effects of interferon. Biochim. biophys. Acta *516:* 231 – 247 (1978).

15 Havell, E. A.; Hayes, T. G.; Vilcek, J.: Synthesis of two distinct interferons by human fibroblasts. Virology *89:* 330 – 334 (1978).

16 Havell, E. A.; Yip, Y. K.; Vilcek, J.: Characteristics of human lymphoblastoid (Namalva) interferon. J. gen. Virol. *38:* 51 – 59 (1977).

17 Isaacs, A.; Cox, R. A.; Rotem, Z.: Foreign nucleic acids as the stimulus to make interferon. Lancet *ii:* 113 – 116 (1963).

18 Isaacs, A.; Lindenmann, J.: Virus interference. I. The interferon. Proc. Roy. Soc., Lond. B *147:* 258 – 267 (1957).

19 Johnson, H. M.; Baron, S.: Interferons: Effects on the immune response and the mechanism of activation of the cellular response. CRC crit. Rev. Biochem. *4:* 203-227 (1976).

20 Johnson, H. M.; Stanton, G. J.; Baron, S.: Relative ability of mitogens to stimulate production of interferon by lymphoid cells and to induce suppression of the in vitro immune response. Proc. Soc. exp. Biol. Med. *154:* 138 – 141 (1977).

21 Kawade, Y.: Purification of murine interferon. Tex. Rep. Biol. Med. *35:* 181 – 186 (1977).

22 Kleinschmidt, W. J.; Cline, J. C.; Murphy, E. B.: Interferon production induced by statalon. Proc. natn. Acad. Sci. *52:* 741 – 744 (1964).

23 Koblet, H.; Wyler, R.; Kohler, U.: Increase of interferon antiviral activity by exogenous adenosine-3'5'-monophosphate (cAMP). Experientia *35:* 575 – 576 (1979).

24 Lakovic, V.; Borecky, L.: Interferon-like and antibody-like substances in mouse peritoneal cells stimulated by myxoviruses in vivo. Acta virol., Prague *9:* 382 (1965).

25 Lee, S. H. S.; van Rooyen, C. E.; Ozere, R. L.: Additional studies of interferon production by human leukemia leukocytes in vitro. Cancer Res. *29:* 645 – 652 (1969).

26 Rotem, Z.; Cox, R. A.; Isaacs, A.: Inhibition of virus multiplication by foreign nucleic acid. Nature *197:* 564 – 566 (1963).

27 Salvin, S. B.; Youngner, J. S.; Lederer, W. H.: Migration inhibitory factor and interferon in the circulation of mice with delayed hypersensitivity. Infect. Immunity *7:* 68 – 75 (1973).

28 Schwarz, L. A.; Fleischmann, W. R., Jr.: (Unpublished observations).

29 Stewart, W. E., II: Interferon nomenclature. Nature *286:* 110 (1980).

30 Stobo, J.; Green, I.; Jackson, L.; Baron, S.: Identification of a subpopulation of mouse lymphoid cells required for interferon production after stimulation with mitogens. J. Immun. *112:* 1589 – 1593 (1974).

31 Strander, H.; Cantell, K.: Production of interferon by human leukocytes in vitro. Ann. Med. exp. Biol. Fenn. *44:* 265 – 273 (1966).

32 Weber, J. M.; Stewart, R. B.: Cyclic AMP potentiation of interferon antiviral activity and effect of interferon on cellular cyclic AMP levels. J. gen. Virol. *28:* 363 – 372 (1975).

33 Wheelock, E. F.: Interferon-like virus-inhibitor induced in human leukocytes by phytohemagglutinin. Science *149:* 310 – 311 (1965).

W. Robert Fleischmann, Jr., PhD, Associate Professor of Microbiology, University of Texas Medical Branch, Dep. of Microbiology, USA- Galveston/TX 77 550

Natural-Killer Cell Activation in Patients Following Human Interferon-Beta Therapy

G. R. Pape[1, 2], *M. R. Hadam*[2], *J. Eisenburg*[1], *G. Riethmüller*[2]

[1] Med. Klinik II, Klinikum Großhadern, München, FRG
[2] Institut für Immunologie, Universität München, FRG

Introduction

Natural-killer (NK) cells are defined by their ability to kill without deliberate prior sensitization of certain tumor cells, virus-infected cells, and normal cells in vitro. During the past few years, increasing evidence supports the importance of these cells both for animals and humans. NK cells are regarded as an important component of the natural resistance to malignancy and to viral infections. Moreover, they are thought to be involved in the homeostasis of certain normal cells.

The elegant studies of *Trinchieri et al.* [21] have demonstrated the key regulatory role of interferon in NK-cell activation in vitro. This experimental observation has provided much support for the new therapeutical approach of administering interferon for certain neoplastic disorders and viral diseases in man. Since to our knowledge of interferon's in vivo effects in man on natural cytotoxicity has been limited to leukocyte interferon [4, 7] and short-term kinetics, it was of particular interest to study its effects on natural-killer cells following long-term application of high doses of human fibroblast interferon (IFN-β).

Material and Methods

Interferon

The interferon used for i.v. injections was human fibroblast interferon (IFN-β) provided by Dr. Rentschler (Rentschler GmbH & Co, Laupheim, Fed. Rep. of Germany). The specific activity of the interferon preparation was 10^6 units/mg protein. IFN-β doses ranged from $1-10 \times 10^6$ units per application. The preparation was found to increase natural cytotoxicity of peripheral blood lymphocytes in a dose-dependent fashion in vitro.

Patients

The study was done on occasion of a controlled trial of IFN-β treatment of patients with chronic hepatitis [15 and *Müller et al*]. NK activity was monitored in 6 patients. The patients were all males, aged 22–44 y.

Lymphocyte Preparation

Nonadherent lymphocytes were isolated from heparinized venous blood by Ficoll-Urovison density centrifugation and then incubated in tissue culture flasks to remove adherent cells.

Preparation of Lymphocyte Subpopulations

T-lymphocytes were identified by their capacity to form rosettes with AET-treated sheep erythrocytes (E_{AET}) [9]. The rosetting fraction was separated from the nonrosetting fraction by centrifugation on a Percoll density gradient [6]. This isolation procedure resulted in a suspension containing 97% E_{AET}-RFC. The rosettes were dissociated by incubation at 37°C for 15 min with frequent vortex mixing. T-cells were separated from E_{AET} by a prewarmed Percoll density gradient [6]. T-cells with Fc receptors for IgG (Tγ) [13] were isolated from the total

T-cell fraction on a Percoll density gradient after rosette formation with bovine erythrocytes coated with rabbit IgG antibodies (E_bIgG) [13, 16]. The erythrocytes were subsequently lysed with distilled water (at 4°C for approximately 15 s).

Cytotoxicity Assay

Cells from the erythroleukemic cell line K562 [12], which is the most sensitive NK target cell described in man [8], were used as target cells in all experiments. The cells were ^{51}Cr labeled and the natural cytotoxicity was measured in a 4 h assay. The test was set up in triplicate samples (variance among triplicates of less than 10%) in tissue culture plates containing 5×10^3 K562 cells and lymphocyte numbers according to the chosen lymphocyte to target cell ratio 12.5:1, 25:1, 50:1, 100:1, respectively, in Parkers' 199+10% fetal bovine serum (FBS) per well. After incubation at 37°C in 95% air +5% CO_2, 0.1 ml of the supernatant was withdrawn and the release of ^{51}Cr was determined by a scintillation counter. The percentage of ^{51}Cr released from the cells, corrected for the maximum release as defined by treatment of target cells by Triton X and for the ^{51}Cr release in lymphocyte-free control tubes ($\geqslant$ 7%), was used as a measure of lysis [17]. Healthy lymphocyte donors were repeatedly tested to ensure the consistency of the assay.

Results

Several charges of human IFN-β were used for this study. Lot Nr. 8 was applied to patients A. K., P. K., M. R., and U. L., who frequently showed side effects such as fever, chills, headache, and muscle pain. Under treatment with a different charge of human IFN-β (Lot Nr. 10), which was used for patients T. M. and R. S., one patient exhibited no side effects except occasional slight headaches. The other patient infrequently showed raised temperature up to 39°C, whereas chills were rare.

Short- and long-term kinetics of NK activity following human IFN-β administration: 4 h after the initial i.v. injection of IFN-β, natural cytotoxic activity was measured in 4 patients (dose of IFN-β $1-4 \times 10^6$ units). As demonstrated in figure 1 a distinct decrease of

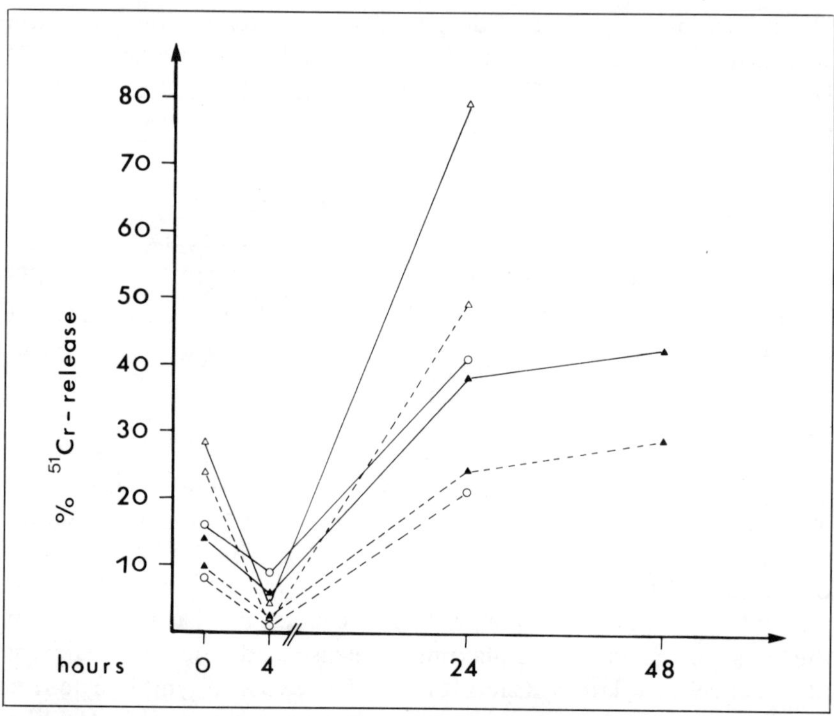

Figure 1. Short-term effects of initial i. v. injection of human IFN-β on NK activity of peripheral blood lymphocytes in patients with HBsAg positive chronic hepatitis. Pat. P. K. (○—○) and pat. M. R. (△—△) after injection of 4×10^6 units; pat. R. S. (▲—▲) after injection of 1×10^6 units. Abscissa: time (h) after interferon injection. Ordinate: percentage ^{51}Cr release from K562-target cells, corrected for release in medium controls ($\leq$ 5%). Solid lines: lymphocyte to target cell ratio (L:T) 50:1 for P. K. and M. R., 100:1 for R. S. Broken lines: L:T 25:1 for P. K. and M. R., 50:1 for R. S.

NK activity was found. After 24 h, cytotoxic activity had increased to 196–282% of pretreatment values. After 48 h, killing activity remained high. Even during peak NK activity, a characteristic short-term decrease was observed after i.v. injection of IFN-β. Simultaneously with the transient fall of cytotoxicity, the absolute and relative numbers of lymphocytes in the peripheral blood decreased (relative percentage of lymphocytes prior to IFN-β injection in pat. T. M. and in pat. R. S. 45%, 4 h after IFN-β injection 8% and 13%, respectively). Absolute numbers of lymphocytes prior to IFN-β injection in pat. T. M. 945, and in pat. R. S. 1530, 4 h after IFN-β injection 448 and 1196, respectively, whereas polymorphonuclear cells (PMN) in-

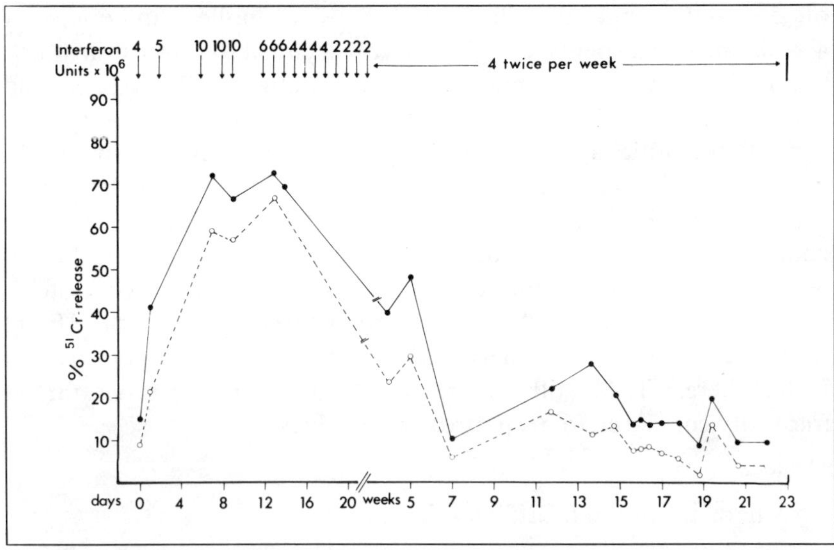

Figure 2. Long-term kinetics of NK activity of peripheral blood lymphocytes in a patient with HBsAg positive chronic hepatitis treated with human IFN-β for several months. Dose of IFN-β (units $\times 10^6$) indicated in graph. Abscissa: time intervals of IFN-β injection. Ordinate: percentage ^{51}Cr release from K562-target cells, corrected for the release in medium controls ($\leqslant$ 5%). Solid line: lymphocyte to target-cell ratio 50:1, broken line: L:T 25:1.

creased. These numbers reflect a transient redistribution of white blood cells (WBC). 24 h after IFN-β injection the numbers had returned to preinjection levels in nearly all instances. The over-all level of WBC was slightly reduced in 2 patients after therapy with IFN-β for 5 weeks (e.g. total WBC prior to IFN-β therapy: pat. T. M. 3400, pat. R. S. 5200; after 5 weeks of IFN-β therapy: pat. T. M. 2100, pat. R. S. 3400, respectively). In the other patients, leukopenia was not observed during long-term human IFN-β therapy.

Figure 2 depicts the results of an in vitro monitoring of natural cytotoxicity in a patient receiving human IFN-β for several months. After a strong augmentation of natural cytotoxicity following the initial injection of IFN-β (the transient fall of natural cytotoxicity usually observed after 4 h is not demonstrated in the graph), the killing activity remained at high levels when IFN-β was given in high doses. Subsequently, the cytotoxic activity decreased when the dose of IFN-β was reduced from $6-2 \times 10^6$ units per day. During a follow-up study of 5 months, during which IFN-β was applied in doses of 4×10^6 units twice per week, NK activity declined to pretreatment levels. Similar results were obtained with two patients, who were treated with high doses of IFN-β (10×10^6 units per day) for 4 weeks. In both patients the initial IFN-β injection (1×10^6 units) caused a manifold increase in NK activity. Also, the cytolytic activity reached peak levels after further application of IFN-β. During 4 repeated 5-day courses of IFN-β, short-term increases of NK activity could be detected after each dose, although the over-all level of natural cytotoxicity seemed to decline. A few days after termination of the IFN-β treatment, natural cytotoxicity reached pretreatment levels in patient R. S., whereas T. M. still demonstrated slightly increased natural cytotoxicity compared to his pretreatment values.

Characterization of Effector Cells

The characterization of the cytotoxic effector cells revealed that the majority expressed Fc receptors for IgG (FcR^+). By density gradient fractionation of lymphocytes forming rosettes with IgG-coated bovine erythrocytes (E_bIgG) most of the activity was recovered in the $E_b IgG^+$ fraction. Thus, the corrected ^{51}Cr release from K562-target cells for patient P. K. was: unfractionated lymphocytes 49.3%, FcR^+ 38.6%, FcR^- 4.9%; patient U. L.: unfractionated lymphocytes 61.8%, FcR^+ 43.7%, FcR^- 6.2% (all values given for effector to target cell ratio of 25:1). The fact that the cytotoxicity was not enriched in the FcR^+ fraction, although this fraction is enriched for FcR^+ NK cells, can be partly explained by the modulation of Fc receptors for IgG on effector cells by the rosetting procedure [16]. When the lymphocytes were separated into T-cells (E-rosette-forming cells, ERFC) and non-T-cells (non-ERFC), cytotoxicity was found in both fractions. The non-T-fraction contained between 3 and 10% ERFC. In the ERFC-population, natural cytotoxicity was expressed by cells with Fc receptors for IgG (Tγ).

Discussion

Activation of NK activity is one of the major mechanisms through which interferon exerts its biological function. Therefore, monitoring of natural cytotoxicity in patients receiving human IFN-β was the prime aim of the presented study. The short-term kinetics of natural cytotoxicity exhibited a characteristic pattern. Injection of IFN-β resulted in a depression of the NK activity of peripheral blood lymphocytes, when tested as early as 2 or 4 h after the administration, irrespective of the actual level of natural cytotoxicity prior to application. This phenomenon was constantly observed except in one instance, where the initial human IFN-β injection enhanced the lytic activity after 4 h. The cause for the constant transient fall of cytotoxicity is presently unknown. The simplest explanation would be transient redistribution of effector cells as seen, for example, after administration of glucocorticoids [5]. Indeed, differential blood counts, performed at the time of decreased natural cytotoxicity, demonstrate an absolute and relative reduction of lymphocyte numbers. Furthermore, this effect was so far not observed after in vitro application of interferon.

The kinetics of augmentation of NK activity during chronic stimulation with human IFN-β revealed following features: (1) the highest relative increase was seen during the initial phase of IFN-β application; (2) at a plateau of high activity, short-term increases after IFN-β injection were much less pronounced; (3) in all patients monitored so far, over a period of several weeks, a gradual decrease of augmented NK activity was observed in spite of continued application of high doses of human IFN-β. At the present time it is difficult to explain these observations, since the activation mechanism of natural cytotoxicity by interferon is unknown. In principle two possible mechanisms, which are not mutually exclusive, have to be considered: (a) a direct activation of the intrinsic lytic potential of NK cells; and (b) a stimulation or recruitment of an initially noncytotoxic NK precursor population. It has been shown that interferon exerts a direct effect on several specialized cell functions, such as increased cytotoxicity of sensitized lymphocytes to allogenic target cells [11, 24] and increased expression of H_2 antigens on the surface of normal lymphocytes [22]. A similar alteration of the expression of surface features by interferon, that might effect the lytic potential of the cells, has to be considered. Recent data [14, 20] suggest that interferon influences the differentiation of active NK cells from inactive precursors. If so, the inability of human IFN-β, at least with the interferon preparation we used and under our therapeutical protocol, to maintain a maximal cytotoxic level could be explained by the "exhaustion" of the pre-NK pool. The actual level of NK activity may be controlled by stimulating factors, such as interferons, and suppressing factors, such as certain prostaglandins [3], as well as by suppressor cells [1]. A dynamic equilibrium of pre-NK and NK cells [10] has been proposed. Continued administration of interferon will shift the balance in one direction. Moreover, in view of a possible homeostatic function on hemopoietic cells [2, 19], potentially harmful effects on hemopoiesis by chronic stimulation of the NK system cannot be excluded.

The active cytotoxic cells revealed features identical to those described for NK cells by others and ourselves [19, 18, 23]: lymphoid cells with Fc receptors for IgG, comprising cells of the T-cell and the non-T-cell lineage.

Our study on natural cytotoxicity was a controlled trial of human IFN-β treatment in patients with HBsAg-positive chronic hepatitis [15, and *Müller et al.*]. The trial is not yet closed. At present it remains to be shown whether the effects of human IFN-β on the course of the disease can be correlated with the induced changes in NK activity. The potentiation of a defense mechanism directed against virus-infected cells in patients with chronic virus infections is noteworthy by itself.

In conclusion, the short-term kinetics of NK activity in patients receiving human IFN-β were similar to those which have been reported for human leukocyte interferon (IFN-α) by *Einhorn et al.* [4] and by *Huddleston et al.* [7]. The long-term kinetics demonstrate that it may be difficult to maintain the initially IFN-β-induced high levels of NK activity during prolonged therapy, at least under our therapeutic regimen. Monitoring of NK activity in patients receiving interferon is, therefore, essential for the development of therapeutic protocols for optimal and sustained augmentation of NK activity in vivo. Such efforts may have important practical implications, since the clinical results of immunotherapy may depend – at least in part – on the effects of NK activity.

Acknowledgments

This study was performed at a multicenter trial of human IFN-β treatment on patients with HBsAg positive chronic active hepatitis, organized by *P.-H. Hofschneider*, (Max Planck-Institut für Biochemie, Martinsried bei München) and *F. Deinhardt* (Max von Pettenkofer-Institut, Universität München), and supported by the FRG Ministry of Research and Technology, Bonn.

We wish to thank Miss *J. Döhrmann* for excellent technical assistance.

This study was supported by Deutsche Forschungsgemeinschaft, Grant Pa 212/3.

References

1 Cudkowicz, G.; Hochman, P. S.: Regulation of natural-killer-cell activity by macrophage-like and other types of suppressor cells. In: Siskind (ed.), Developmental Immunology – Fifth Irwin Strasburger Memorial Seminar on Immunology (Grune and Stratton, New York 1978).

2 Cudkowicz, G.; Hochman, P. S.: Do natural-killer cells engage in regulated reactions against self to ensure homeostasis? Immunol. Rev. *44*: 13–41 (1979).

3 Droller, M. J.; Schneider, M. U.; Perlmann, P.: A possible role of prostaglandins in the inhibition of natural and antibody-dependent cell-mediated cytotoxicity against tumor cells. Cell. Immunol. *39:* 165–177 (1978)

4 Einhorn, S.; Blomgren, H.; Strander, H.: Interferon and spontaneous cytotoxicity in man. II. Studies in patients receiving exogenous leukocyte interferon. Acta med. scand. *204*: 477–483 (1978).

5 Fauci, A. S.: Glucocorticoid effects on circulating human mononuclear cells. J. reticuloendoth. Soc. *26:* 727–738 (1979).

6 Feucht, H. E.; Hadam, M. R.; Frank, F.; Riethmüller, G.: Improved separation of human peripheral T-cells using PVP-coated colloidal silica particles (Percoll). In: Peters (ed.), Separation of cells and subcellular elements, pp. 73–76 (Pergamon Press, Oxford – New York 1979).

7 Huddlestone, J. R.; Merigan, T. C., Jr.; Oldstone, M. B. A.: Induction and kinetics of natural-killer cells in humans following interferon therapy. Nature *282:*417–419 (1979).

8 Jondal, M.; Pross, H.: Surface markers on human B- and T-lymphocytes. VI. Cytotoxicity against cell lines as a functional marker for lymphocyte subpopulations. Int. J. Cancer *15:* 596–605 (1975).

9 Kaplan, M. E.; Clark, C.: An improved rosetting assay for detection of human T-lymphocytes. J. immunol. Methods *5:* 131–135 (1974).

10 Kiessling, R.; Hochman, P. S.; Haller, O.; Shearer, G. M.; Wigzell, H.; Cudkowicz, G.: Evidence for a similar common mechanism for natural-killer-cell activity and resistance to hemopoietic grafts. Eur. J. Immunol. *7:* 655–663 (1977).

11 Lindahl, P.; Leary, P.; Gresser, I.: Enhancement by interferon of the specific cytotoxicity of sensitized lymphocytes. Proc. natn. Acad. Sci. *69:* 721–728 (1972).

12 Lozzio, C. B.; Lozzio, B. B.: Cytotoxicity of a factor isolated from human spleen, J. natn. Cancer Inst. *50:* 535–538 (1973).

13 Moretta, L.; Ferrarini, M.; Mingari, M. C.; Moretta, A.; Webb, S. R.: Subpopulations of human T-cells identified by receptors for immunoglobulins and mitogen responsiveness. J. Immun. *117:* 2171–2174 (1976).

14 Oehler, J. R.; Herberman, R. B.: Natural cell-mediated cytotoxicity in rats. III. Effects of immunopharmacologic treatments on natural reactivity augmented by polyinosinic-polycytidylic acid. Int. J. Cancer *21:* 221–229 (1978).

15 Pape, G. R.; Hadam, M. R.; Eisenburg, J.; Hofschneider, P.-H.; Riethmüller, G.: Natürliche Zytotoxizität beim Menschen: Stimulation in vivo durch Interferon. In: Vhdlg. Dtsch. Ges. Innere Med., Vol. 86, pp. 1454–1457 (J. F. Bergmann, München 1980).

16 Pape, G. R.; Moretta, L.; Troye, M.; Perlmann, P.: Natural cytotoxicity of human Fc-receptor positive T-lymphocytes after surface modulation with immune complexes. Scand. J. Immunol. *9:* 291–296 (1979).
17 Pape, G. R.; Troye, M.; Axelsson, B.; Perlmann, P.: Simultaneous occurrence of immunoglobulin-dependent and immunoglobulin-independent mechanisms in natural cytotoxicity of human lymphocytes. J. Immun. *122:* 2251–2260 (1979).
18 Pape, G. R.; Troye, M.; Perlmann, P.: Characterization of cytolytic effector cells in peripheral blood of healthy individuals and cancer patients. II. Cytotoxicity to allogeneic or autochtonous tumor cells in tissue culture. J. Immun. *118:* 1925–1930 (1977).
19 Peter H. H.; Pavie-Fischer, J.; Fridman, W. H.; Aubert, C.; Cesarini, J. P.; Roubin, R.; Kourilsky, F. M.: Cell-mediated cytotoxicity in vitro of human lymphocytes against a tissue culture melanoma cell line (IGR3). J. Immun. *115:* 539–547 (1975).
20 Saksela, E.; Timonen, T.; Cantell, K.: Human natural-killer activity is augmented by interferon via recruitment of "pre-NK" cells. Scand. J. Immunol. *10:* 257–266 (1979).
21 Trinchieri, G.; Santoli, D.: Antiviral activity induced by culturing lymphocytes with tumor-derived or virus-transformed cells. Enhancement of human natural – killer-cell activity by interferon and antagonistic inhibition of susceptibility of target cells to lysis. J. exp. Med. *147:* 1314–1333 (1978).
22 Vignaux, F.; Gresser, I.: Differential effects of interferon on the expression of H-2K, H-2D, and Ia antigens on mouse lymphocytes. J. Immun. *118:* 721–727 (1977).
23 West, W. H.; Cannon, G. B.; Kay, H. D.; Bonnard, G. D.; Herberman, R. B.: Natural cytotoxic reactivity of human lymphocytes against a myeloid cell line: Characterization of effector cells. J. Immun. *118:* 335–361 (1977).
24 Zarling, J. M.; Sosman, J.; Eskra, L.; Borden, E. C.; Horoszewicz, J. S.; Carter, W. A.: Enhancement of T-cell cytotoxic responses by purified human fibroblast interferon. J. Imm. *121:* 2002–2004 (1978).

Dr. med. Gerd R. Pape, Med. Klinik II, Klinikum Großhadern, Postfach 701260, D-8000 München 70

Host Genotype Influences Interferon Action in the Mouse

Jaqueline De Maeyer-Guignard, Françoise Dandoy, Edward De Maeyer

Institut Curie, Université de Paris-Sud, Orsay, France

Introduction

In addition to host genes controlling levels of interferon production in response to some viruses [9], there is increasing evidence for host genes influencing interferon action. The study of such genes should not only provide a better understanding of the basic mechanisms involved in the interaction of interferons and cells, but also help to explain the pronounced individual variations in the reaction to interferon treatment observed in some clinical trials [2]. Indeed, the existence of different alleles at loci, influencing the efficacy of interferon action, could represent one of the many factors implicated in the individual response to interferon treatment. In our opinion, this rather unexplored area merits more attention than it has received so far.

The best characterized locus influencing interferon activity is situated on the long arm of chromosome 21 in man; it affects the antiviral and cell multiplication inhibitory activity of α and β interferons. Human cells, trisomic for chromosome 21, are more sensitive to both these effects of interferon, and, moreover, peripheral blood monocytes from subjects with trisomy 21 show a 3.7-fold increased sensitivity to the maturation-inhibiting effect of interferon [3, 5, 11, 12, 20, 21]). Although good indirect evidence suggests that the locus on human chromosome 21 codes for interferon receptors, a definite demonstration is still lacking [18, 19]. A corresponding locus, *If-rec*, has recently been mapped in the mouse on chromosome 16 [4, 15].

In normal diploid individuals or cells, no differences in interferon action have been attributed to the existence of different alleles at these loci; as already mentioned, the presence of an extra gene copy seems to be necessary to enhance sensitivity to interferon action. However, it is probably not too far-fetched to predict that such alleles will eventually be found.

A very interesting example of a gene influencing interferon activity was recently provided by *Haller et al.* Mice of the A2G-strain have been known for a long time to be resistant to what in most mice would be a lethal infection with influenza A virus and this resistance is determined by a single dominant locus, *Mx* [16]. It was recently shown that this locus specifically and exclusively affects interferon sensitivity of orthomyxo virus replication; these viruses are much more efficiently inhibited by interferon in *Mx/Mx* cells than they are in +/+ cells. This differential effect is not observed with other viruses [14].

Our own work deals with differences in interferon action that can be observed between mice belonging to two inbred strains, BALB/c and C57BL/6. The main reason for employing animals of these 2 strains is the existence of seven recombinant inbred and many congenic lines, derived from them by *Bailey,* facilitating genetic analysis and linkage studies [1]. In addition, both the parental strains and the lines developed from them have been well characterized for interferon production with several viruses, which enables us to look for possible linkage of genes influencing interferon production and action. In this short review we summarize some of our findings concerning mouse genotype and interferon action.

Experimental Results

While studying immunomodulation by interferon of delayed-type hypersensitivity (DH) in the mouse, we observed significant differences in the reaction to interferon between BALB/c and C57BL/6 mice [10]. When interferon is given 24 h before immunization with sheep erythrocytes (SRBC), inhibition of sensitization is more pronounced in BALB/c mice than in C57BL/6 mice. When it is given only 1 h before SRBC, inhibition of sensitization no longer occurs in C57BL/6 mice whereas it is still significant in BALB/c mice. Thus,

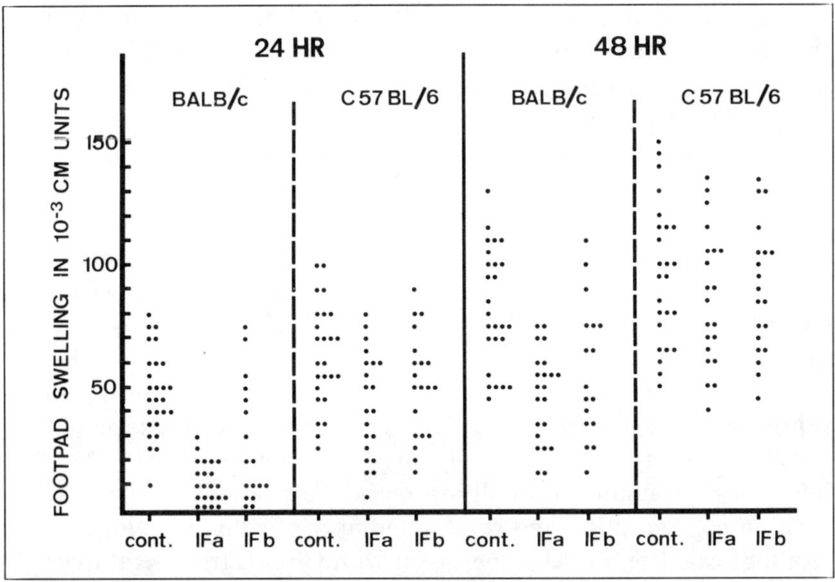

Figure 1. Immunosuppressive effect of interferon on expression of DH to SRBC in BALB/c and C57BL/6 mice. The results of three different experiments are combined. Three-month-old female BALB/c and C57BL/6 mice were sensitized by an i.v. inoculation of 10^6 SRBC. Four days later and 3 h before footpad challenge, the interferon-treated group received an i.p. inoculation of 1 ml containing 3.3×10^5 interferon units (IFa), 3.3×10^4 interferon units (IFb) or phosphate-buffered saline (cont.). Footpad swelling was measured 24 h (a) and 48 h (b) after challenge. Each point represents the footpad swelling of one mouse (with permission from [10]).

the immunosuppressive effect of exogenous interferon on the afferent pathway of DH to SRBC is more pronounced in BALB/c than C57BL/6 mice. A difference between mice of the two genotypes is also observed when the influence of interferon on the expression of DH to SRBC is examined. When given a few hours before footpad challenge, interferon inhibits the expression of DH in both strains. However, it is less active in C57BL/6 mice. For example, a dose leading to a pronounced inhibition of footpad swelling in sensitized BALB/c mice remains without significant effect in C57BL/6 mice. About 25 times the amount of interferon used in BALB/c mice is needed to obtain comparable inhibition of footpad swelling in C57BL/6 mice (fig. 1). These observations suggested that, in addition to having different alleles at genes influencing the production of interferon, BALB/c and C57BL/6 mice have also different alleles at loci influencing the action of interferon on cells of the immune system, and we therefore looked for other possible differences in interferon action between these two mouse strains. As a result of this, it has become evident that the greater sensitivity of the BALB/c genotype to interferon action is also expressed when the cell multiplication inhibitory effect is examined. This was demonstrated using two different cell types, committed erythroid precursors and bone-marrow-derived macrophages. In the presence of electrophoretically pure interferon graded at 5 antiviral units per ml, the number of colonies obtained from erythropoietin-stimulating cultures of C57BL/6-marrow cells is hardly, or not at all, reduced in comparison with controls, whereas colony counts from BALB/c or Swiss cells consistently show inhibition of 30 to 40% [13]. The difference between the two types of response subsists with increasing interferon concentrations, but becomes less pronounced. In all instances, the relationship between interferon concentration and residual number of colonies is linear on a semilog scale (fig. 2). An experiment with CFU-E from fetal liver instead of bone marrow has confirmed this strain dependence of sensitivity to interferon, in that again cells of BALB/c genotype are more sensitive to inhibition by interferon [13].

When the effect of interferon on the development of bone-marrow-derived macrophages in culture is examined, a similar picture emerges [6]. Proliferation of marrow-derived cells is inhibited by interferon and the effect is dose dependent, confirming previously published work of others [17, 22]. Again, proliferation of BALB/c cells is more readily inhibited than is proliferation of C57BL/6 cells, the difference in susceptibility being about 5-fold (fig. 3). Macrophages from the congenic B6-C-H-2^d mice have a sensitivity to the cell multiplication inhibitory effect of interferon which is comparable to that of cells derived from C57BL/6 mice, and this would seem to rule out an effect of genes in the major histocompatibility complex [6]. Lack of linkage to the MHC was also found when committed erythroid precursors instead of macrophages were studied.

All the foregoing observations point to the existence of genes influencing the degree of sensitivity to interferon action, with BALB/c mice having the alleles determining the higher sensitivity. Inhibition of cell proliferation and of delayed hypersensitivity are non-antiviral activities of interferon, and the relevant question was whether the BALB/c genotype also determined an enhanced sensitivity to the an-

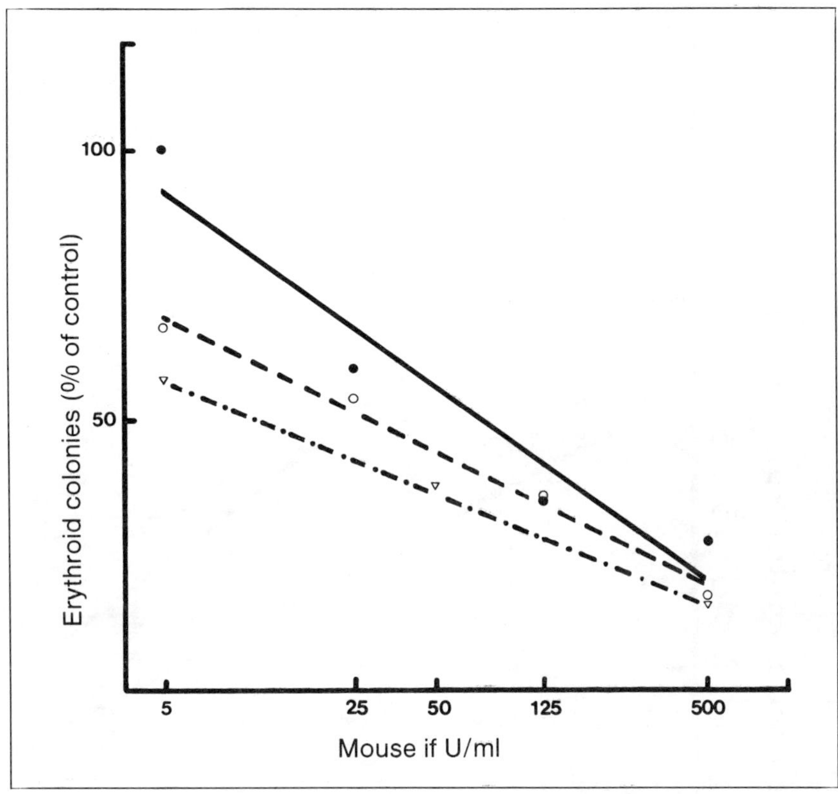

Figure 2. Strain dependence of the inhibitory effect of pure mouse interferon on bone-marrow erythroid colony formation. Each regression line is calculated from the results of 7 separate experiments. (●) C57BL/6, slope – 36, with a standard deviation from the regression line of 8.3%. The values for the Swiss and BALB/c strains are (O) Swiss, –25, 2.5%, and (Δ) BALB/c, –20.7, 1.6%. Electrophoretically pure mouse interferon derived from C-243 cells induced with Newcastle disease virus was used. The specific activity of the preparation used was $2x10^9$ NIH reference units per mg of protein, in good agreement with our previously published value. Analysis by polyacrylamide gel electrophoresis on slab gel showed only the 2 interferon bands previously described. All experiments were carried out with a single interferon preparation with a titer of 64,000 units per 0.2 ml, which was distributed into 0.1-ml portions and stored frozen at –70°C. When used, the portion was thawed and further diluted in DMEM. Sheep plasma erythropoietin (step 3, lot 3019-6, 15 IRP units per mg; Connaught Medical Laboratories) was used (with permission from [13]).

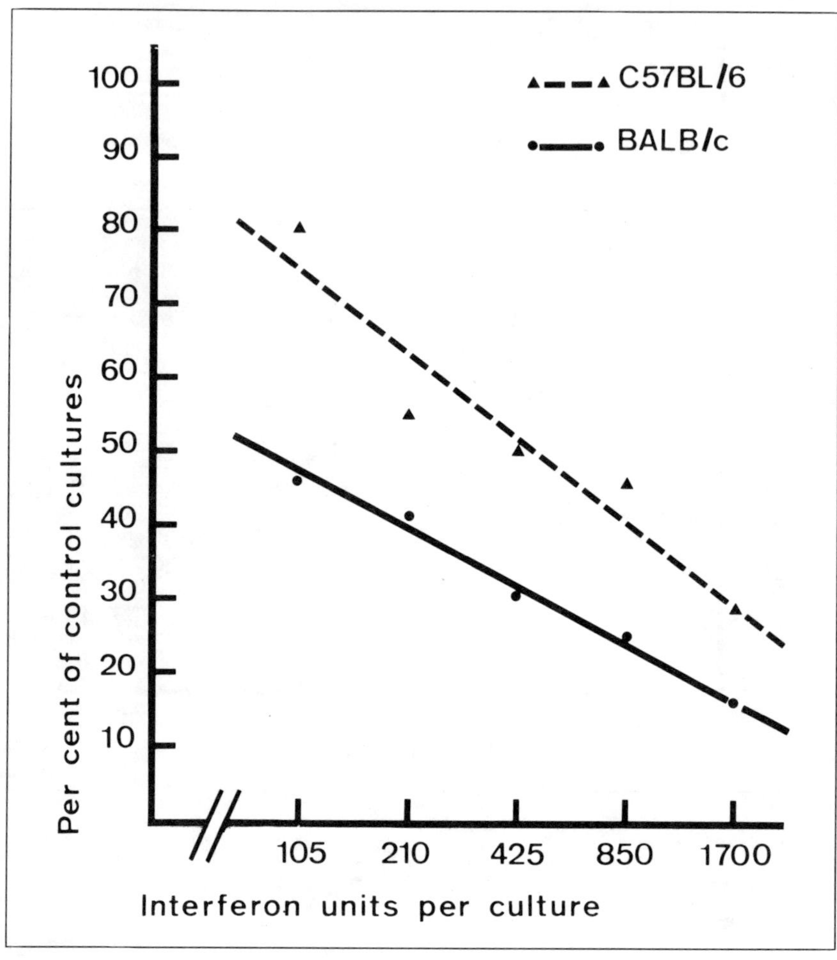

Figure 3. Dose-response curves of the cell multiplication inhibitory effect of interferon on bone-marrow-derived cells in culture. Each point represents the average of four cultures, expressed as % of control cultures, counted on day 5 after onset of culture. The two regression lines were calculated according to the least squares method. The average cell number in the 4 C57BL/6 control cultures was 1.40×10^5, and in the BALB/c cultures 1.25×10^5 (with permission from [6]).

tiviral action of interferon. This has been examined by comparing the protective effect of exogenous interferon on a lethal infection with encephalomyocarditis virus (EMCV) in BALB/c and C57BL/6 mice.

In EMCV-infected mice, interferon treatment results in a better protection of BALB/c than of C57BL/6 mice, and, for example, a single inoculation of $6x10^5$ units of interferon brings about a more prolonged survival and decreased final mortality of BALB/c mice [7]. Evidently, as with the immunomodulating and the cell multiplication inhibitory effect of interferon, the BALB/c genotype is also responsible for an enhanced sensitivity to the antiviral effect of interferon. However, the protection conferred by interferon to BALB/c and C57BL/6 embryo fibroblast cultures infected with EMCV does not reflect the difference observed in vivo, since in tissue culture BALB/c fibroblasts are not more sensitive to the antiviral action of interferon than C57BL/6 fibroblasts [8]. We are currently trying to establish in which cells the genes affecting interferon action are expressed.

Discussion

For every interferon activity that has been examined, immunomodulation in vivo, inhibition of cell multiplication in vitro, and antiviral action in vivo, the BALB/c genotype determines the greater sensitivity. We believe it a reasonable assumption that we are dealing with the effect of the same gene(s) in all three cases, but have so far no evidence to substantiate this. In this respect, it will be most interesting to compare levels of the different enzymes activated by interferon in cells of BALB/c and C57BL/6 genotype, since this could be a common denominator for all effects that were examined.

Two lines of evidence indicate that the *If-rec* locus is not directly involved in the genetic differences described in the present paper. First, from analogy with the human situation as regards chromosome 21, only mice trisomic for *If-rec* would be expected to have enhanced sensitivity to interferon [3, 5, 11, 12, 20, 21] and the animals used in our work are normal diploid mice; however, as discussed in the introduction, we cannot formally excude that we are measuring the effect of different alleles at the *If-rec* locus in BALB/c and C57BL/6 mice. A second argument against involvement of the *If-rec* locus is the fact that, contrary to the effects described in this paper, one would expect the *If-rec* locus to be expressed in fibroblasts in vitro [4, 15]. We have not found a difference either in the antiviral or in the cell multiplication inhibitory effect of mouse interferon when tested in embryo fibroblast cultures derived from BALB/c and C57BL/6 mice (*Dandoy et al.*, unpublished observation). Evidently, not all cells express the different interferon sensitivities of the two genotypes. Since in vitro the enhanced sensitivity of BALB/c cells has been observed in cultures of committed erythroid precursors and of bone-marrow-derived macrophages, we think it possible that the greater sensitivity of the BALB/c genotype to interferon action may principally be expressed in cells derived from the hemopoietic system, such as lymphocytes or macrophages. This will be examined in more detail in further experiments.

We would like to recall here that, in the case of interferon induction with some viruses, C57BL/6 mice are high and BALB/c mice low interferon producers [9]. The intriguing possibility that the high interferon production of C57BL/6 mice is related to the decreased sensitivity of some C57BL/6 cells to interferon action should be considered and will be explored since it may have physiological implications. One could indeed speculate that in high interferon producers, a decreased sensitivity of some cells to interferon might be a desirable feature, since it would protect these cells against possible untoward effects of interferon, such as, for example, depression of bone-marrow function during viral infections.

Acknowledgments

Aided by a grant from the Fondation pour la Recherche Médicale, the CNRS (AI 031858) and the DGRST (allocation d'étude du troisième cycle).

We thank *Dr. D. W. Bailey* of the Jackson Laboratory at Bar Harbor, Maine (USA) for providing us with the congenic and recombinant inbred strains used in this study.

References

1 Bailey, D. W.: Recombinant inbred strains. An aid to finding identity, linkage, and function of histocompatibility and other genes. Transplantation *11:* 325–327 (1971).

2 Borden, E. C.: Personal communication. As a result of the ongoing clinicals trials with interferon organized by the American Cancer Society, it is the definite impression of the investigators that there exist groups of individuals showing different sensitivities to the biologic effects of interferon.

3 Chany, C.; Vignal, M.; Couillin, P.; Nguyen van Cong; Boue, J.; Boue, A.: Chromosomal localization of human genes governing the interferon-induced antiviral state. Proc. natn. Acad. Sci. USA *72:*3129–3133 (1975).

4 Cox, D. R.; Epstein, L. B.; Epstein, C. J.: Genes coding for sensitivity to interferon (If-rec) and soluble superoxide dismutase (SOD-1) are linked in mouse and man and map to mouse chromosome 16. Proc. natn. Acad. Sci. USA *77:* 2168–2172 (1980).

5 Cupples, C. G.; Tan, Y. H.: Effect of human interferon preparations on lymphoblastogenesis in Down's syndrome. Nature *267:*165–167 (1977).

6 Dandoy, F.; De Maeyer, E.; De Maeyer-Guignard, J.: Antiproliferative action of interferon on murine bone-marrow-derived macrophages is influenced by the genotype of the marrow donor. J. Interferon Res. *1:*263–270 (1981).

7 Dandoy, F.; De Maeyer-Guignard, J.; De Maeyer, E.: Mouse genotype influences the antiviral activity of interferon. In: De Maeyer, Galasso, Schellekens (eds.), The Biology of the Interferon System, pp. 197–200 (Elsevier, Amsterdam, 1981).

8 Dandoy, F.; De Maeyer-Guignard, J.; Bailey, D.; De Maeyer, E.: Mouse genes influence antiviral action of interferon in vivo (submitted for publication).

9 De Maeyer, E.; De Maeyer-Guignard, J.: Considerations on mouse genes influencing interferon production and action. In: Gresser (ed.), Interferon 1979, pp. 75–100 (Academic Press, London 1979).

10 De Maeyer, E.; De Maeyer-Guignard, J.: Host genotype influences immunomodulation by interferon. Nature *284:*173–175 (1980).

11 Epstein, L. B.; Epstein, C. J.: Localization of the gene AVG for the antiviral expression of immune and classical interferon the distal portion of the long arm of chromosome 21. J. infect. Dis. *133:*A 56–A 62 (1976).

12 Epstein, L. B.; Lee, S. H. S.; Epstein, C. J.: Enhanced sensitivity of trisomy 21 monocytes to the maturation-inhibiting effect of interferon. Cell. Immunol. *50:* 191–194 (1980).

13 Gallien-Lartigue, O.; Carrez, D.; De Maeyer, E.; De Maeyer-Guignard, J.: Strain dependence of the antiproliferative action of interferon on murine erythroid precursors. Science *209:*292–293 (1980).

14 Haller, O.; Arnheiter, H.; Lindenmann, J.; Gresser, I.: Host gene influences sensitivity to interferon action selectively for influenza virus. Nature *283:*660–662 (1980).

15 Lin, P. F.; Slate, D. L.; Lawyer, F. C.; Ruddle, F. H.: Assignment of the murine interferon sensitivity and cytoplasmic superoxide dismutase genes to chromosome 16. Science *209:*285–287 (1980).

16 Lindenmann, J.; Lane, C. A.; Hobson, D.: The resistance of A2G mice to myxoviruses. J. Immun. *90:*942–951 (1963).

17 McNeill, T. A.; Gresser, I.: Inhibition of haemopoietic colony growth by interferon preparations from different sources. Nature new Biol. *244:*173–174 (1973).

18 Revel, M.; Bash, D.; Ruddle, F. H.: Antibodies to a cell-surface component coded by human chromosome 21 inhibit action of interferon. Nature *260:* 139–141 (1976).

19 Slate, D. L.; Ruddle, F. H.: Antibodies to chromosome 21-coded cell surface components can block response to human interferon. Cytogenet. Cell Genet. *22:* 265–269 (1978).

20 Tan, Y. H.; Tischfield, J.; Ruddle, F. H.: The linkage of genes for the human interferon-induced antiviral protein and indophenol oxidase-B traits to chromosome G-21. J. exp. Med. *137:*317–330 (1973).

21 Tan, Y. H.; Schneider, E. L.; Tischfield, J.; Epstein, J.; Ruddle, F. H.: Human

chromosome 21 dosage: Effect on the expression of the interferon-induced antiviral state. Science *186:* 61 – 63 (1974).

22 Van't Hull, E.; Schellekens, H.; Lowenberg, B.; De Vries, M. J.: Influence of interferon preparations on the proliferative capacity of human and mouse bone-marrow cells in vitro. Cancer Res. *38:* 911 – 914 (1978).

Jaqueline De Maeyer-Guignard, MD, Institut Curie, Université de Paris-Sud, Campus d'Orsay – Bat. 110, F-91504 Orsay

A Monoclonal Antibody against Interferon-Alpha

D. C. Burke

University of Warwick, Department of Biological Sciences, Coventry, Great Britain

This study, which was done in collaboration with *Dr. David Secher* in Cambridge, was initiated about 4 years ago and has led to the isolation of a monoclonal antibody to interferon-α [1].

Basically the technique of monoclonal-antibody formation is one for immortalizing an antibody-producing cell. The antibody response is normally heterogeneous in terms of the antigens that are injected, the antigenic site on the molecule, and also the antibody that is formed. The discovery by *Kohler* and *Milstein* [2] of the technique of monoclonal-antibody formation provides a way of immortalizing the antibody-producing cell. The technique depends upon cell fusion. Immortal myeloma cells, which grow continuously in culture, are fused with the spleen cells from the immune animal. From the hybrid cells which are formed, those are selected which produce antibody for the antigen in question. One can formally compare this process to that of gene cloning, because both involve the formation of a bank of hybrid cells, followed by a difficult, and often tedious process of screening these new cells for either the production of a new antigen (in monoclonal antibody formation) or a new gene (in gene cloning). The spleen cells are fused with the myeloma cells, plated out into wells under conditions that ensure that only hybrid cells will survive and grow. These hybrid cells are then screened for the formation of a specific antibody. These antibody-producing cells can be grown in vitro or in the mouse. The antibody produced by these cells is always the same, directed against a single antigenic site. Since the cells have arisen from a single fusion event, they are, by definition, monoclonal.

The mice were injected with partially or more highly purified preparations of lymphoblastoid interferon and the antibody titer was followed as a function of time after injection. BALB/c mice were injected every two weeks with interferon and then the antibody titer was measured one week after each infection. There was considerable variation between the mice in the response but antibody titers did not rise beyond 3 and 4 $\log_{10}$. That has been a consistent observation whether we used this material or the much more crude material which we used in an earlier series of experiments. It is difficult to decide at what point to fuse. Clearly, if there are no antibody-forming cells in the spleen, it is a waste of time fusing, but, in fact, the only parameter one has is the antibody titer in the circulation. This responds rather slowly and, clearly, the optimal time will be when B-cells are maximally active inside the spleen rather than at the maximum activity of circulating antibody titer. In our case, we followed the circulating anti-interferon titer in the serum until the values ceased to rise and fused at that point. We then screened selected hybrid cells for the production of an anti-interferon. Since the antigen that we injected had not been pure, we could not use an antibody-binding technique for screening, but a neutralization technique. This meant that the supernatant fluids from the hybrid cells were mixed with interferon and the resulting titer was measured. For this purpose, we needed a precise and reliable interferon assay.

We used an assay with which we have considerable experience, that is the use of Semliki Forest virus as a challenge virus and the virus growth was measured by incorporating radioactive uridine into viral RNA in the infected cells. Pretreatment of the cells with interferon reduces the amount of viral growth, the amount of viral RNA synthesis, and therefore the counts which are incorporated. We were looking for an anti-interferon effect, and for an increase in counts as a mark of the antibody titer.

Figure 1 shows a result of an early screen. The hybrid cells were plated out into 48 wells and the supernatant fluids were tested at

---

Figure 1. Screening of cell culture supernatant fluids for anti-interferon activity by the direct method. Culture fluid was mixed with about 2 international units of lymphoblastoid interferon, added to HFF cells which, after overnight incubation, were challenged with Semliki Forest virus. Virus growth was measured as ^{3}H-uridine incorporation into intracellular virus RNA. The incorporation in the presence of interferon alone is shown by the dotted line, and the incorporation in the absence of interferon (the virus control) was double this value. The lines show the effect on viral RNA synthesis of mixing with cell culture fluids harvested 13 days (top panel), 16 days (middle panel), and 20 days (bottom panel), after the fusion (with permission from [5]).

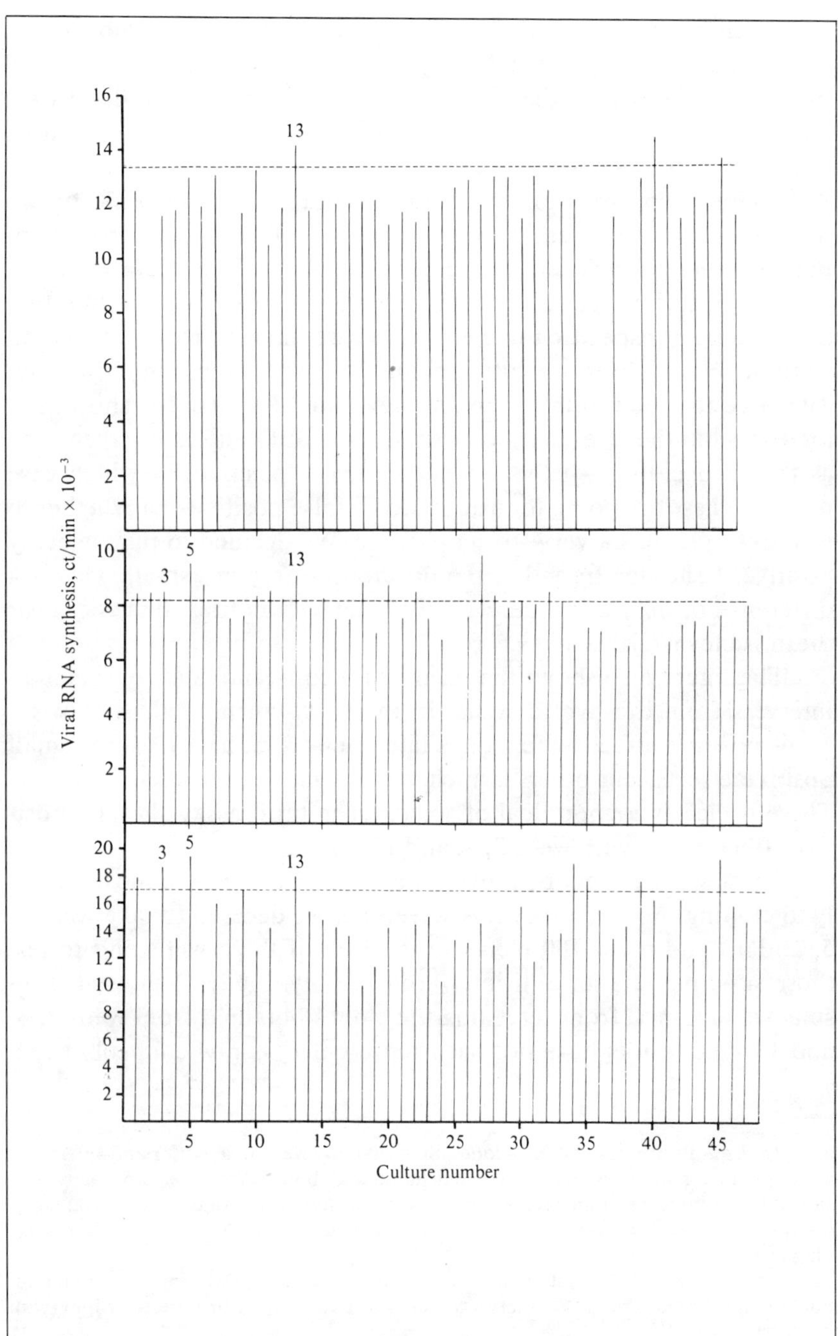
Viral RNA synthesis, ct/min × 10⁻³
Culture number
13
3
5
13
3
5
13

about one-weekly intervals. The vertical axis shows the radioactivity, which is a mark of viral RNA synthesis, and the horizontal dotted line shows the counts that will be expected if interferon alone were added to the human cells. This is the effect of the interferon dose (1 unit) which was mixed with the tissue culture fluids.

There is considerable variation around this figure. First of all, there are some supernatant fluids where the effect of interferon is apparently increased. There is less viral RNA synthesis than expected and the interferon effect appears to be augmented. We assume that this is some nonspecific toxic effect, but we have no real information about it. What we are actually looking for is an increase in radioactivity above that due to interferon alone. A number of wells show such increases but the effects are very small. The difficulty in a screen such as this is deciding whether to pursue every positive, in which case many of these are going to turn out to be false positives, or whether to wait until one has a very strong positive. We decided to pursue every positive. I should stress that the differences are very small. This is a difference of only a few percent of the interferon titer. It is very near the noise level of this assay.

The figure also shows the results of 3 consecutive assays taken at intervals from the hybrid wells. In the first screen, well 13 shows a small positive effect. A few days later wells 3, 5, and 13 show small positive effects, but others, which were negative before, are positive. There is clearly a good deal of scatter. The third assay shows a positive effect, again with wells 3, 5, and 13.

These wells cannot be grown indefinitely. One has to move quickly to cloning. As a result of this screening, we decided to take wells 3, 5, and 13 and grow 100 clones from each of these wells and to test those supernatants for anti-interferon activity. Figure 2 shows the results we obtained from screening the clones obtained from wells 3, 5, and 13. The results have not been represented as raw counts but as a

---

Figure 2. Properties of NK2-clones. Supernatants were assayed for anti-interferon activity and for the presence of secreted immunoglobulin. Anti-interferon activity is shown by an increase in the level of RNA synthesis above that due to interferon alone (– –). Secreted Ig was detected by a reverse plaque assay.

Open circles (○) indicate that the supernatants were negative for secreted immunoglobulin; closed circles (●) that they were positive (a, b, c) or untested (d, e) (with permission from [1]).

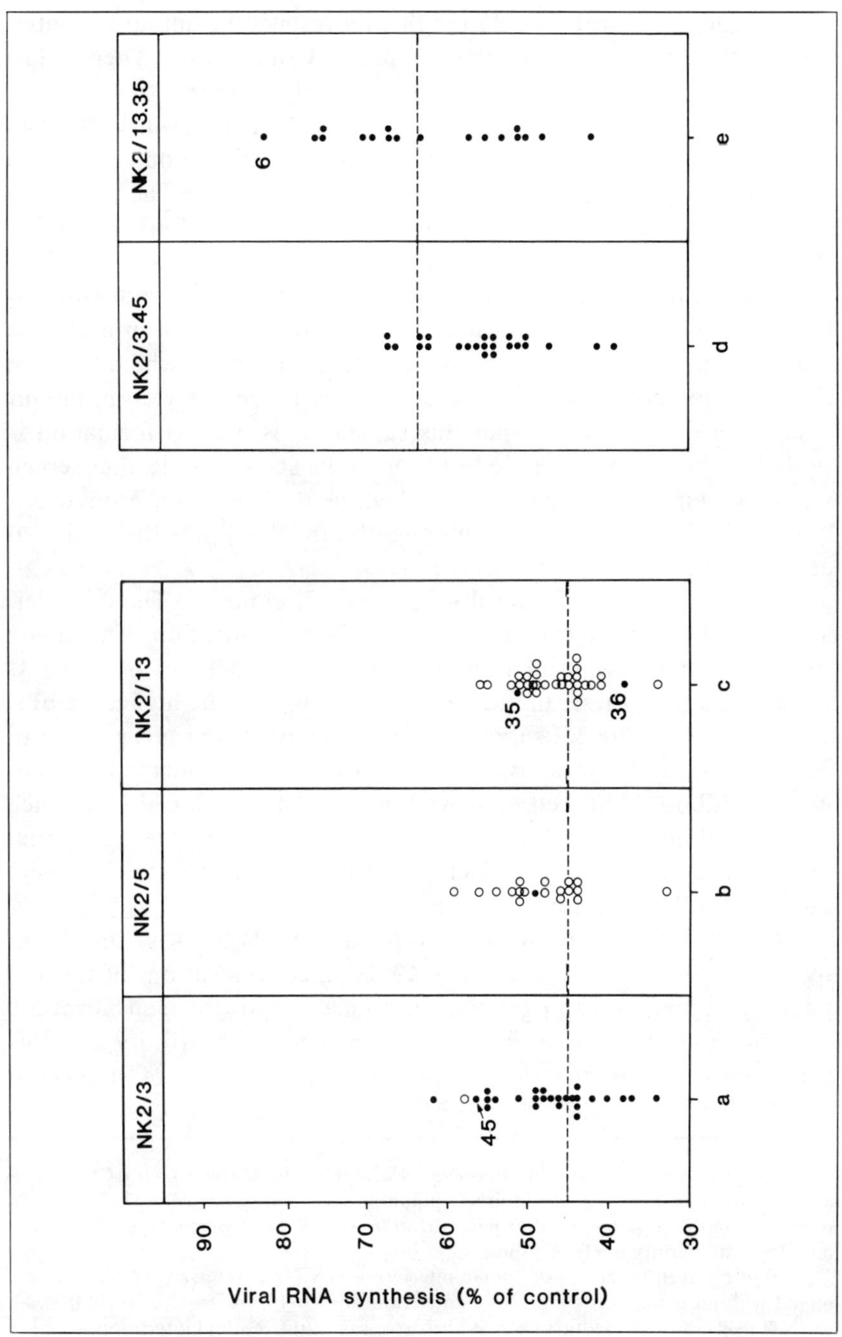
NK2/3
NK2/5
NK2/13
NK2/3.45
NK2/13.35
45
35
36
6
a
b
c
d
e
90
80
70
60
50
40
30
Viral RNA synthesis (% of control)

percentage of control. The dotted line represents the amount of interference that is due to the interferon mixed with the fluid. There is just over one unit of interferon, depressing the virus control to just under 50%. Figure 2 shows the results of mixing the supernatant fluids from clones obtained from well 3 with that dose of interferon. There is a scatter of responses ranging from 60% down to 40%. The same was obtained from clones in wells 5 and 13. We selected clone 45 for further study from well 3, and clone 35 and 36 from well 13.

This figure, in which circles are filled, shows cells producing immunoglobulin whereas all others failed to produce any in a reverse plaque test. Some clones were producing a substance which was not an immunoglobulin but appeared to neutralize interferon in our assay. We do not know what this substance is, but its formation is probably the reason we failed in a previous screening. In that screen we isolated a clone, like this one, which neutralized interferon activity but failed to release any immunoglobulin. Work was discontinued at that point.

Panel (d) shows that results from well 3, clone 45. The considerable scattered results do not show much neutralization. The figure (panel e) shows the results obtained with the subclones of clone 35 from well 13. Of these, the subclone 6, which gave the highest results, was selected. Clone 35, subclone 6 was a clone called NK2 and produced anti-interferon activity. From NK 2 we obtained the monoclonal antibody. This cell grew well in mice and produced IgG which neutralized interferon. A large number of other clones were potential anti-interferon antibody formers but for logistical reasons we were unable to follow these up.

Figure 3 shows the neutralization of lymphoblastoid interferon by the IgG obtained from clone NK2. High concentrations of IgG (10 μg/ml) are necessary in order to produce significant neutralization. This suggests that the antibody is not of very high affinity and this was confirmed by the dose-response curves (fig. 4) of interferon

Figure 3. Neutralization of IFN-α by NK2-IgG as measured by either the direct anti-interferon assay (○) or the indirect immunoprecipitation assay (●). The interferon remaining in the supernatant after neutralization is shown as a percentage of the original titer (with permission from [5]).

Figure 4. Neutralization of human interferon-α by NK2. Interferon dilutions were mixed with an equal volume of NK2 antiserum diluted 10^{-1} (○—○), 10^{-2} (◆—◆), 10^{-3} (■—■), or with medium (▲—▲) before assay of the residual interferon.

% IFN
remaining
in supernatant
100
90
80
70
60
50
40
30
20
10
0
1
10
100
[IgG] μg/ml

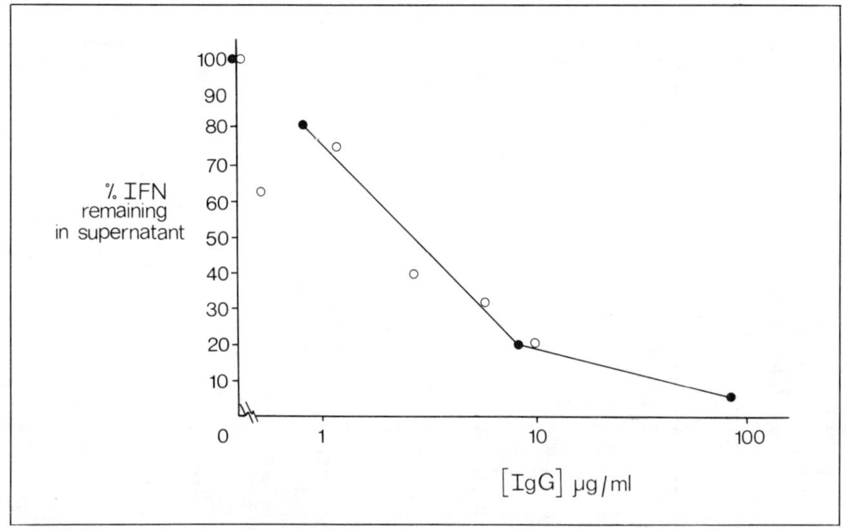

3

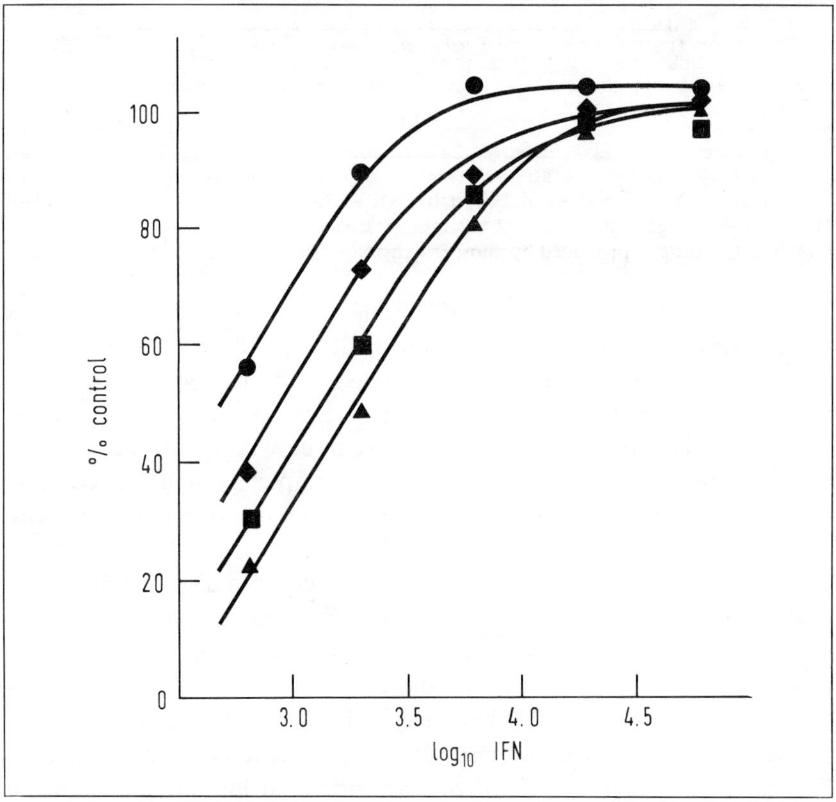

100
80
60
40
20
0
% control
3.0
3.5
4.0
4.5
log10 IFN

4

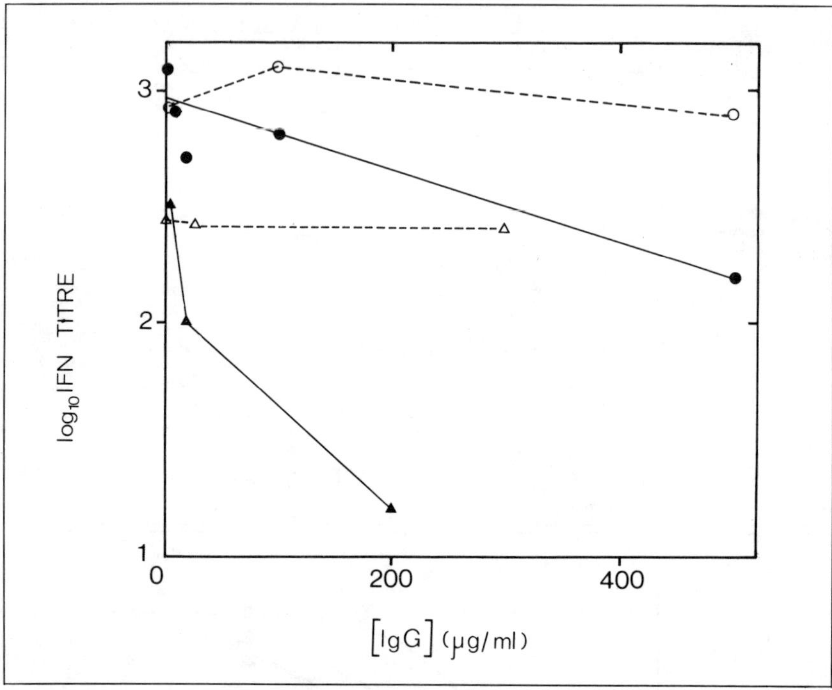

Figure 5. Neutralization of IFN-α by NK2-IgG (▲) or by W6/32 (△), and of IFN-β by NK2-IgG (●) or by W6/32 IgG (○). W6/32 is an IgG directed against a human HLA antigen produced by another hybrid cell (with permission from [5]).

mixed with differing dilutions of the antibody. The RNA synthesis is depicted as a percent of control, a measure of virus yield, using different interferon dilutions. The triangles show the effect of interferon alone; this is a typical dose-response curve. When the interferon is mixed with antibody, it is partially or completely neutralized. The maximum effect is obtained with a 10^{-1} of the dilution antibody. The neutralization is less with a 10^{-2} dilution and, at a 10^{-3} dilution, it cannot be detected. This should be compared with a polyclonal antibody which will dilute out to 10^{-5} and still produce a neutralizing effect. *Y. Kawada* [3] points out that the existence of such parallel dose-response curves argues for an antibody with low affinity. Despite this low affinity, however, it has been useful for a number of purposes.

First of all we were interested in the specificity of this material. Figure 5 shows the effects of this antibody on human interferon-β.

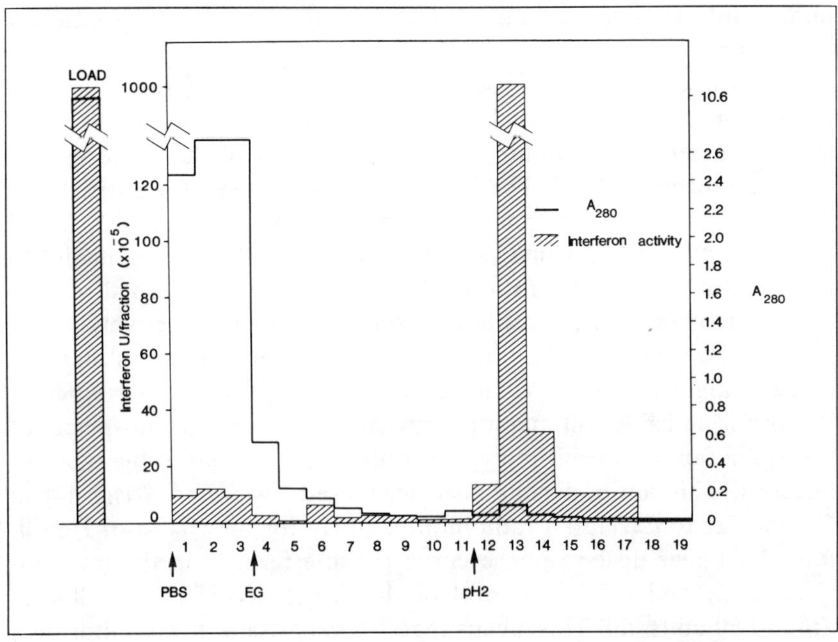

Figure 6. Affinity chromatography of partially purified lymphoblastoid interferon. Lymphoblastoid interferon (10^8 U, 0.5 ml PBS, 1.9×10^7 U/mg) was loaded onto a 0.5 ml NK2-Sepharose column. Fractions of 0.5 ml were collected. The column was washed successively with PBS; 9.1 M ethanediol, 0.34 M NaCl, 0.114 M Na-phosphate buffer pH 7.4 ("EG"); 9.1 M ethanediol, 0.3 M NaCl, 0.1 M citric acid ("pH 2") as indicated. Fractions were assayed for interferon content and for protein content by measuring A_{280} and assuming an $E_{280}^{1\%}$ of 10 (with permission from [1]).

There are two neutralizations shown here, one by the anti-interferon monoclonal antibody NK2 and one by a monoclonal derived from another clone, which is completely irrelevant to the present work. These materials, as the IgG, were mixed at varying concentrations with a dose of interferon-β that titrated at 3 $\log_{10}$ in the interferon assay. This is about 1000 units of interferon. The irrelevant supernatant had no effect at all, but there is a possible reduction in interferon titer at 500 μg/ml of IgG, while there is no reduction at 100 μg of IgG/ml, the difference from the control titer being not significant in the assay. Thus the highest concentration appeared to have a small effect on interferon-β, but using a column of the IgG-absorbed to Sepharose we were not able to retain any interferon-β. We conclude that this small neutralizing effect is non-specific. The antibody does not neutralize human interferon-β or mouse interferon. It seems to be specific for interferon-α.

All these experiments use a mixture of the interferon-α species. At the time, we did not realize how extensive the alpha family was. We are currently determining exactly how many of the alpha species are neutralized by NK2. The antibody has been used for purification (fig. 6). A small column, containing about 7 mg of the antibody which had been partially purified, was washed with PBS and ethanediol to remove nonspecific absorption. The interferon is deabsorbed right at the front of the pH 2 profile and the recovery is effectively 100%. Some interferon, the bulk of proteins, and a small amount of material come straight through. We are currently trying to discover whether this last is an irrelevant material or whether it is a minor subspecies of the alpha family since it represents only a few percent of the total interferon. This antibody has also been used by *David Secher* [4] in Cambridge to develop a radioimmunoassay for interferon-α. He obtained a linear dose-response curve for interferon-α in the radioimmunoassay and the lower level of the sensitivity of this method is around 50 units/ml. This means that it is very useful for monitoring a purification process and in procedures where large amounts of interferon are being formed. It is still not suitable for monitoring the rather small amounts of interferon that are formed in patients' response to viral infection and to other treatments. We probably need a more avid antibody or a combination of more than one monoclonal antibody. Clearly this antibody can be used for both purification and estimations of interferon and we hope it will prove to be useful in the coming years.

References

1 Secher, D. S.; Burke, D. C.: A monoclonal antibody for large-scale purification of human leukocyte interferon. Nature *285:* 446–450 (1980).

2 Kohler, G.; Milstein, C.: Continuous cultures of fused cells secreting antibody of predefined specificity. Nature *256*: 495–497 (1975).

3 Kawada, Y.: An analysis of neutralization reaction of interferon by antibody: A proposal on the expression of neutralization titer. J. Interferon Res. *1:* 61–70 (1980).

4 Secher, D. S.: Immunoradiometric assay of human leukocyte interferon using monoclonal antibody. Nature *290:* 501–503 (1981).

5 Morser, J.; Meager, A.; Burke, D. C.; Secher, D. S.: Production and screening of cell hybrids producing a monoclonal antibody to human interferon-α. J. gen. Virol. *53:* 257–265 (1981).

Prof. Dr. D. C. Burke, University of Warwick, Dept. of Biological Sciences,
GB-Coventry CV4 7AL, Warwickshire

Monoclonal Antibodies against Human Fibroblast Interferon

H. K. Hochkeppel, U. Menge, J. Collins

Gesellschaft für Biotechnologische Forschung mbH, Braunschweig, FRG

Introduction

Monoclonal antibodies are superior to conventional antibodies because of their unique specificity to a single antigenic determinant and because of their high titers and constant yields [1, 2, 3]. In the case of interferon, so far only one report has described the successful isolation of a hybridoma line secreting mouse monoclonal antibodies to human leukocyte interferon [4]. We have now established a stable hybrid myeloma line (FO) which secretes antibodies against human fibroblast interferon. Since interferon is known to be a potent antiviral agent and is also regarded as a potential antitumor agent [5], monoclonal antibodies against human fibroblast interferon will be very helpful for assaying human IFN-β expression of DNA cloned in *E. coli* or for efficient large-scale purification of the protein with a monoclonal antibody column. We established a stable hybridoma line which secretes monoclonal IFN-β antibodies by neutralizing the antiviral activity of human IFN-β as opposed to human IFN-α and by the Elisa-assay technique as well as by specific immunoadsorption of IFN-β to a monoclonal antibody column.

Material and Methods

Cell line: The mouse myeloma line FO, used for fusion experiments with mouse spleen lymphocytes, was a gift of Hans Trachsel from the Friedrich Miescher-Institut, Basel. The line is a variation of the myeloma line SP2/0 and was originally established by *Groth and Scheidegger* [6].

Media: Myeloma cells were cultured in IMDM (Gibco), 10% FCS, and hybrid-myeloma in HAT-IMDM, 20% FCS.

Immunization of mice: Purified IFN-β [7] was injected into 8-week-old female Balb/c mice. Injections were carried out at weekly intervals with 1 μg IFN-β per mouse. Mice, having a titer of IFN-antibodies which inhibited human IFN-β in a direct antiviral assay [8] at a serum dilution ratio of 1:200, were chosen for lymphocyte fusion experiments. Four days before spleen excision, a final booster injection with 1 μg IFN-β, from which the sugar part had been removed by treatment with a mixture of sugar degrading enzymes, was administered.

Fusion procedure: The fusion of myeloma (FO) and spleen cells was carried out according to *Köhler and Milstein* [1] with the modification that a feeder layer was omitted. Instead, the hybrids were grown in HAT-medium containing 1% methylcellulose.

Isolation of hybridoma cells which secrete monoclonal anti-IFN-β: Individually growing hybridoma colonies were picked with sterile capillaries after two weeks and cloned separately in costar tissue plate wells. The hybridoma colonies were then tested for inhibition of antiviral activity of IFN-β on FS4 fibroblasts in an indirect antiviral assay according to *Secher and Burke* [4], since the direct antiviral IFN-β assay was not sensitive enough to detect the small amounts of antibodies secreted by primary hybrid cultures. Positive cultures were subcloned, grown for four days and tested with the Elisa-microtiter assay according to *Towbin et al.* [9] as well as with the direct antiviral IFN-β assay. Cultures, which were positive for antibody secretion in both the Elisa and the antiviral assay, were subcloned once more and the supernatant of these cultures again tested in the direct antiviral IFN-β assay [8]. In this way, a stable hybridoma line secreting monoclonal IFN-β antibodies was established.

Indirect antiviral IFN-β assay: The assay was performed on human FS4-cells according to *Secher and Burke* [4] using VSV as challenge.

Direct antiviral IFN-β assay: The assay was performed on human FS4-cells according to *Havell and Vilcek* [8] using VSV as challenge.

Purification of human IFN-β: Crude human IFN-β was purchased from Rentschler and purified over an aqueous 2-phase polyethylene glycol-phosphate system in which the IFN-β is trapped in the upper phase and the bulk of the proteins in the lower phase [7]. The specific activity of IFN-β after a single extraction step was about 7×10^6 units/mg protein, that is a yield of about 90%. The IFN-β material was either precipitated out of this system with 4% perchloric acid or adsorbed by Blue-Sepharose. Purified human leukocyte interferon (IFN-α) was a generous gift of Harald Mohr (Red Cross, Hannover).

Elisa-test: The microtiter Elisa-assay for the identification of monoclonal interferon antibody secreting hybridoma clones was performed as follows: Each well of polyvinyl-Elisa-plate was coated with 50 mg of purified IFN-β. After saturating all unspecific binding sites with 3% BSA, supernatant of hybridoma cultures was added for 16 h at room temperature. Then peroxidase-conjugated rabbit anti-mouse IgG was added at a dilution ratio of 1:500 in tris-buffered saline, 5% horse serum, and 0.5% BSA for 2 h at room temperature and, after a washing step, peroxidase-conjugated goat anti-rabbit-IgG was added (also 1:500 dilution ratio). Color reaction was carried out with 5-aminosalicylic acid as substrate according to *Towbin et al.* [9].

SDS-gel electrophoresis of crude IFN-β and electrophoretic transfer onto a nitrocellulose sheet with subsequent Elisa reaction: Electrophoresis was performed according to Laemmli [10]. The gel was then soaked in a buffer containing 50 mM NaCl, 2 mM Na-EDTA, 4 M urea, 0.1 mM dithiothreitol, 10 mM tris-HCl, pH 7.0, according to *Bowen et al.* [11] and the proteins (IFN-β as well as markers) were electrophoretically transferred onto a nitrocellulose sheet [9]. While the section of the blot containing the markers was stained with amido black, the part containing IFN-β was soaked for 4 h at 37°C in 3% BSA/TBS (tris-buffered saline) to saturate all unspecific protein-binding sites for Elisa. After a washing step in TBS, the purified monoclonal anti-IFN-β IgM was added at a 1:50 dilution ratio in 5% horse serum (containing 0.5% BSA and 0.01% NaN_3) for 16 h at room temperature). After a further washing step in TBS, the blot was then soaked for 2 h in a rabbit-antimouse peroxidase-conjugated IgG solution (1:500 dilution ratio in 5% inactivated horse serum, 0.5% BSA), washed again, and then soaked for another 2 h in a goat-antirabbit peroxidase-conjugated IgG-solution (1:500 dilution ratio as above) to make the Elisa reaction more sensitive. After a final wash, the color reaction was performed with O-dianisidin as substrate. Marker proteins were ovalbumin (45 K) and myoglobin (17.5 K).

Purification of monoclonal anti-IFN-β and coupling of the antibody to CNBr-activated Sepharose: Monoclonal antibodies against IFN-β were purified by a 35% ammoniumsulfate precipitation step with following separation over a Sephadex-G-200 column in a tris-glycine buffer, pH 7.6, containing 0.04% n-butanol. The purified antibodies were then coupled to CNBr-activated Sepharose-4B in a buffer containing 0.1 M $NaHCO_3$ and 0.5 M NaCl at pH 8.3 for 2 h at room temperature. The antibody was then washed with ethanolamine and stored in TBS.

Iodination of IFN-β: The iodination was performed with ^{125}I according to *Hunter et al.* [12].

Immunoadsorption of ^{125}I-IFN-β to the monoclonal antibody column, SDS-gel electrophoresis, and autoradiography: An ^{125}I-labeled crude IFN-β sample was loaded on the column and immunoadsorbed in tris-buffered saline, pH 7.4. A subsequent neutral thorough wash (3 ×) with tris-buffered saline at pH 7.4 removed unspecifically adsorbed protein material. Specifically bound ^{125}I-IFN-β was then washed off the column with 0.1 M glycine/HCl buffer, pH 2.3. The eluted sample was lyophilized and then electrophoresed on an SDS-gel according to *Laemmli* [10] together with non-purified ^{125}I-IFN-β and ^{14}C-labeled protein markers. After electrophoresis the gel was first soaked twice 10 min in DMSO and subsequently for 20 min in DMSO/30% PPO, washed with H_2O, and dried down. The dried gel was then autoradiographed.

Results

Hybridoma colonies, having been subcloned in HAT-medium, were tested for specific anti-IFN-β secretion in an "indirect" antiviral IFN-β assay on human FS4 cells according to *Secher and Burke* [4]. The regular assay system according to *Havell and Vilcek* [8] was not sensitive enough to detect initial antibody secretion. The first table shows an example of positive (i.e. specific anti-IFN-β secreting) cultures detected in this way. The average inhibition of IFN-β by the hybridoma supernatants in comparison to an antibody-free IFN-β control was in the range of 50 – 60%. Hybridoma colonies, revealing weaker inhibition capacity, were frozen away and negative colonies were discarded. Positive hybridoma colonies were then subcloned

Table I. Indirect antiviral assay. Anti-interferon activity of monoclonal antibody containing supernatants of individual hybridoma cultures in the indirect antiviral IFN-assay on FS4-cells with VSV as challenge.

Costar plate well No.	Units IFN-β/ml	% Inhibition
57	1536	60
58	1536	60
59	2048	46.5
60	1072	72.1
69	1792	53.4
70	1792	53.4
Control	3084	0

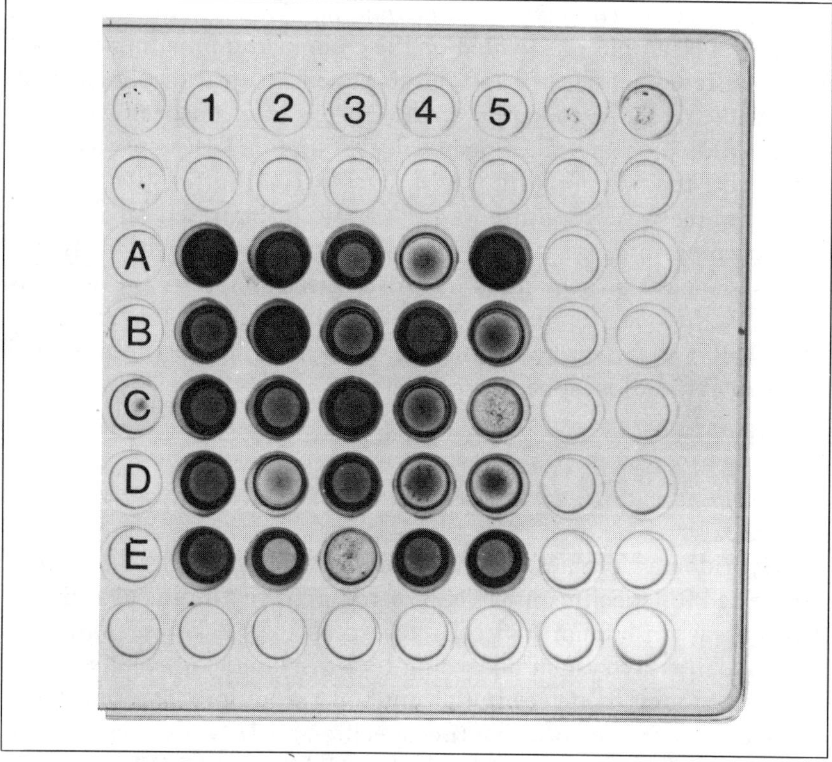

Fig. 1. Microtiter Elisa-assay for the identification of monoclonal-interferon antibody-secreting hybridoma clones. Color reaction was carried out with 5-aminosalicylic acid as substrate according to *Towbin et al.* [9]. A1 – E5 represent an example of different subcloned hybridoma colonies tested for specific antibody secretion.

Table II. Titration of anti-interferon activity of monoclonal antibody containing supernatants of hybridoma cultures. The supernatants were tested at various dilutions for monoclonal antibody activity against IFN-β in the direct antiviral IFN-assay on human FS4-fibroblasts with VSV as challenge.

Concentration of antibody sample	Antiviral activity of standard IFN-β (%)
1 : 3	20
1 : 6	40
1 : 10	70
1 : 20	90
Control, no antibodies	100

again. This was necessary at this early stage of hybridoma culturing, because many hybrid cells still tend to lose their genes, and only a part of the hybridomas eventually stabilizes. Therefore, among the positive cultures, one has to select stable lines. Stable cultures were selected with the Elisa microtiter technique (fig. 1) and then tested once more for specific antibody secretion in the direct antiviral IFN-β-assay according to *Havell and Vilcek* [8].

Figure 1 illustrates an example of the Elisa. The dark, actually brown, wells represent positive hybridoma cultures. The dye intensity was measured at 410 nm against a negative control.

Table II shows the inhibition rate of one of the stable lines in the direct antiviral assay. At a dilution ratio of hybridoma supernatant of 1:3, a maximum of 80% inhibition in comparison to an IFN-β-control is achieved; and at a dilution ratio of 1:20, one still observes a 10% inhibition effect. In general, using individual hybridoma supernatants, only a partial inhibition of the antiviral IFN-β activity was observed. The next step was to demonstrate the specificity of the monoclonal anti-IFN-β. In order to have enough antibodies for the following assays, ascites tumors were grown by injecting the hybridomas (10^6 cells per mouse) into the peritoneal cavity of mice. After removing the cells of the harvested ascites fluid by centrifugation, the monoclonal antibodies were purified by a 35% ammoniumsulfate and a following Sephadex-G-200 column step.

Figure 2 demonstrates that the monoclonal anti-IFN-β is an IgM molecule because it possesses an identical elution profile to an IgM control sample. The purified anti-IFN-β-IgM was then tested for the inhibition of several IFN-β and -α samples (table III). In comparison to an antibody-free IFN-β control, the IgM (diluted 1:30) was able to

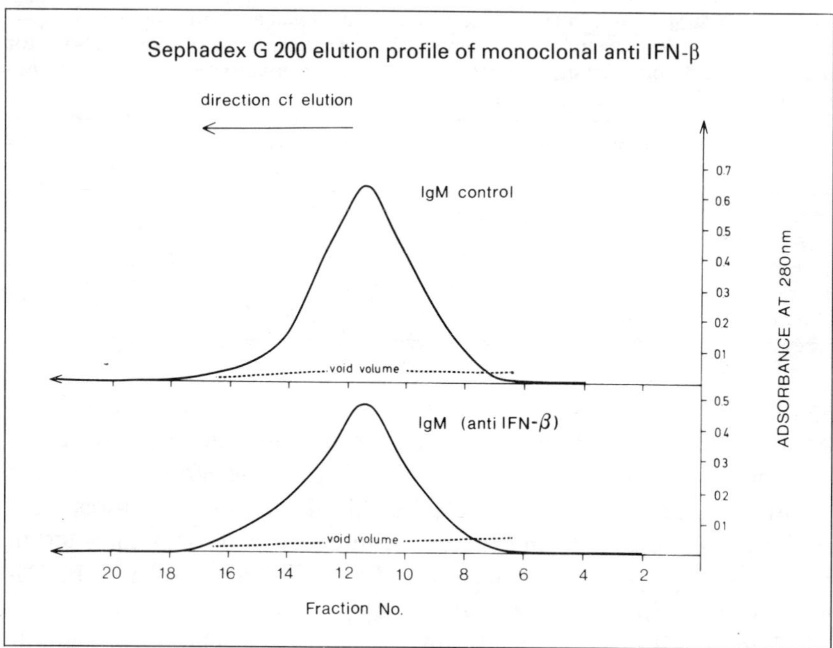

Fig. 2. Sephadex-G-200 elution profile of purified anti-IFN-β in comparison to an IgM-control.

Table III. Inhibition activity of purified monoclonal anti-IFN-β IgM in the direct antiviral assay on FS4-fibroblasts using IFN-β, IFN-β after sugar degradation, and IFN-α.

Concentration of monoclonal IFN-β antibody sample from ascites	Antiviral activity of standard IFN-β (%)
1 : 3	0
1 : 6	0
1 : 30	0
1 : 60	30
1 : 100	80
IFN-β control	100

completely inhibit either the antiviral activity of the complete IFN-β or of an IFN-β sample, which had been treated with a mixture of sugar-degrading enzymes (neuramidase, α-glucosidase, α-manosidase, α/β-galactosidases). Therefore, the monoclonal anti-IFN-β is very likely directed against the protein moiety of IFN-β. After treatment of

Table IV. Titration of ascites fluid for monoclonal anti-IFN-β activity in the direct antiviral IFN-assay on human FS4-cells. Mice, having been pretreated with Freund's adjuvants, were injected with 10^6 hybridoma cells in the peritoneal cavity. After 2-3 weeks, ascites fluids were collected and cells removed by centrifugation.

Sample	% Antiviral protection of FS4-cells
IFN-β (complete molecule), control	100
IFN-β (protein moiety), control	100
IFN-β (complete molecule) plus monoclonal anti-IFN-β	0
IFN-β (protein moiety) plus monoclonal anti-IFN-β	0
IFN-β (complete molecule) plus monoclonal anti-IFN-β (pretreated with trypsin)	100
IFN-β (protein moiety) plus monoclonal anti-IFN-β (pretreated with trypsin)	100
IFN-α control	100
IFN-α plus monoclonal anti-IFN-β	100

the IgM sample with trypsin followed by inhibition of the reaction with soya-bean inhibitor, the inhibition activity of anti-IFN-β in the antiviral assay is destroyed, demonstrating that the inhibition activity is indeed due to a protein, to the monoclonal anti-IFN-β IgM molecule. Also no cross-reaction of anti-IFN-β with human leukocyte interferon (IFN-α) is observed (again table III). After addition of anti-IFN-β to an IFN-α sample, the antiviral activity of IFN-α is unimpaired. This also excludes the possibility that the inhibition of the antiviral activity of IFN-β is due to a protease activity. The purified monoclonal anti-IFN-β IgM was then tested for the inhibition of IFN-β in the direct antiviral assay on FS4-cells at various dilutions of the monoclonal IgM (table IV). At a dilution ratio of the IgM of 1:30, the inhibition is still complete; and a partial inhibition is still observed at an IgM-dilution ratio of 1:100. Next, a crude sample of IFN-β was electrophoresed on an SDS-gel according to *Laemmli* [10] parallel with molecular weight markers (myoglobin, MW 17.5 K, ovalalbumin, MW 45 K). The proteins were then electrophoretically transfered onto a nitrocellulose sheet according to *Towbin et al.* [9]. While the section with the markers was stained, an Elisa-test was performed with the section containing the transfered IFN-β sample.

Figure 3 demonstrates that out of the crude IFN-β sample only one sharp band at about 19 K reacts very specially with the monoclonal anti-IFN-β. To further demonstrate the specificity of the monoclonal anti-IFN-β, a crude IFN-β sample, having been iodinated

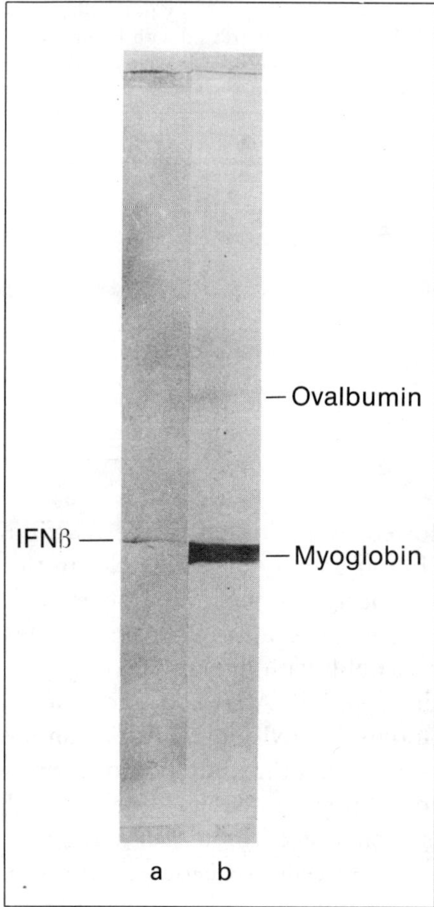

Fig. 3. Electrophoretic transfer of IFN-β from an SDS-gel onto nitrocellulose sheet and subsequent Elisa reaction.
(a) IFN-β (Elisa), (b) Molecular weight standards stained with amido black. Electrophoresis was performed according to *Laemmli.* The proteins (IFN-β as well as markers) were electrophoretically transfered onto a nitrocellulose sheet. While the section of the blot containing the markers was stained with amido black, an Elisa was performed with the blot section containing IFN-β. Color reaction was performed with O-dianisidin as substrate. Marker proteins were ovalbumin (45 K) and myoglobin (17.5 K).

before with ^{125}I according to *Hunter et al.* [12], was tested for specific immunoadsorption to a monoclonal anti-IFN-β-Sepharose column (see material and methods). The immunoadsorbed ^{125}I-IFN-β was then electrophoresed on an SDS gel parallel with non-purified ^{125}I-IFN-β and ^{14}C-protein markers.

Figure 4 illustrates the autoradiograph of the SDS-gel which demonstrates that the column-coupled anti-IFN-β IgM very effectively binds IFN-β. After 4 days of exposure, there is also a very weak second band of higher molecular weight showing up in the autoradiograph. This could be a cross-reacting subclass of IFN-β, since there are indications that possibly 2 or more IFN-β genes exist [13, 14].

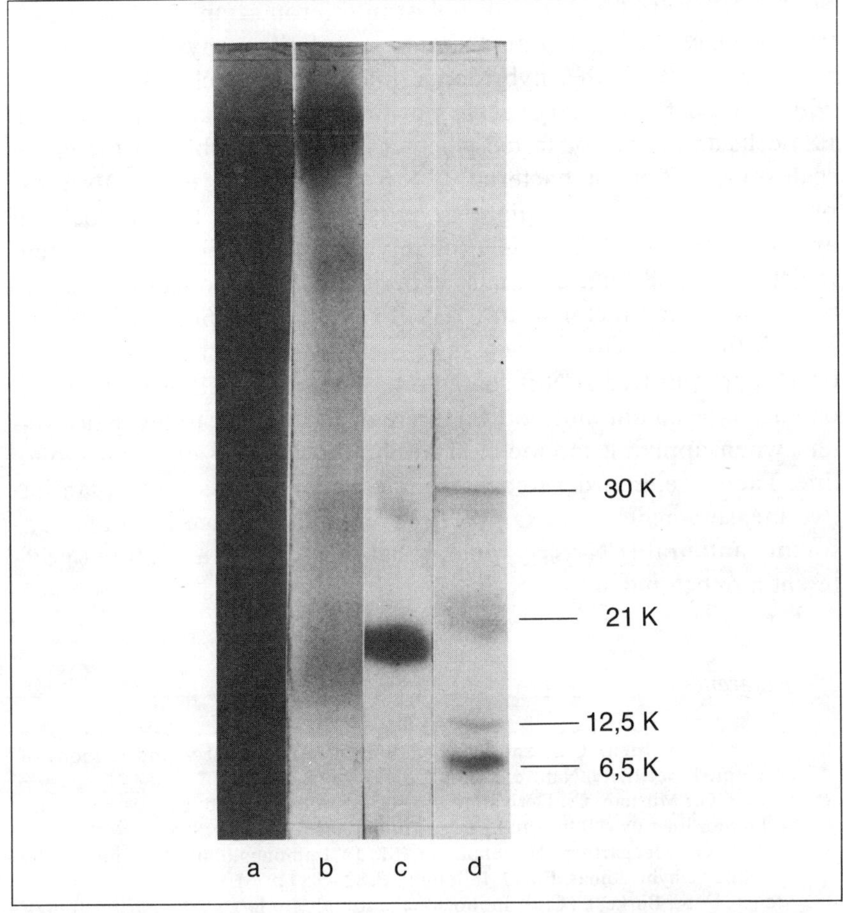

Fig. 4. Autoradiograph of an SDS-gel with (a) nonpurified ^{125}I-IFN-β (4 days exposure), (b) nonpurified ^{125}I-IFN-β (1 day exposure), (c) immunoadsorbed ^{125}I-IFN-β (4 days exposure) and (d) ^{14}C-protein markers (30 K = carbonic anhydrase, 21 K = trypsin inhibitor (soya bean), 12.5 K = cytochrom C, 6.5 K = aprotinin).

Discussion

We have established several stable mouse hybridoma lines which secrete monoclonal human anti-IFN-β. Specificity assays were demonstrated for one of the lines showing that the particular monoclonal anti-IFN-β antibody is an IgM-molecule which can specifically bind IFN-β out of a crude fibroblast interferon sample. In the meantime, we have also performed similar specificity assays for monoclonal anti-IFN-β of other hybridoma lines. The monoclonal antibodies will be used for the large-scale purification of natural IFN-β from FS4-cells and it will be tested whether it is also suitable for the large-scale purification of bacterial IFN-β (i.e. cloned IFN-β-DNA expressed in *E. coli*). This might be possible, because the monoclonal antibody described here is probably directed against the protein moiety of IFN-β. In preliminary experiments we have set up an Elisa-test with the monoclonal anti-IFN-β on polyvinyl-microtiter plates. Even if the sensitivity of the assay system is very high (one can detect 0.002 ng of purified IFN-β coated on a microtiter well using two peroxidase-labeled anti-antibodies), there is no linearity in the assay system when applying monoclonal antibodies of only one hybridoma line. Therefore, in order to achieve linearity of the assay for quantitative measurements, for example to eventually replace the time-consuming antiviral IFN-assay, one probably has to use a mixture of different monoclonal anti-IFN-βs.

References

1 Köhler, G.; Milstein, C.: Continuous cultures of fused cells secreting antibody of predefined specificity. Nature, Lond. *256:*495–497 (1975).
2 Köhler, G.; Milstein, C.: Derivation of specific antibody-producing tissue culture and tumor lines by cell fusion. Eur. J. Immunol. *8:*82–88 (1978).
3 Köhler, G.; Hengartner, H.; Shulman, M. J.: Immunoglobulin production by lymphocyte hybridomas. Eur. J. Immunol. *8:*82–88 (1978).
4 Secher, D. S.; Burke, C. C.: A monoclonal antibody for large-scale purification of human leukocyte interferon. Nature, Lond. *285:*446–450 (1980).
5 Stewart W. E., II; In: The interferon system: Antitumor activities of interferon in animals, pp. 292–320 (Springer, Berlin, Heidelberg, New York 1979).
6 Groth, F. de S. E.; Scheidegger, S.: Production of monoclonal antibodies: Strategy and tactics. J. immunol. Methods *35:*1–25 (1980).
7 Menge, U.; Morr, M.; Anastassiadis, K.; Kula, M. R.: Verfahren zur Reinigung von Interferon. German patent application No. P 2943016.8.
8 Havell, E. A.; Vilcek, J.: Production of High-Titered Interferon in Cultures of Human Diploid Cells. J. antimicrob. Chemother. *2:*476–484 (1972).
9 Towbin, H.; Staehelin, T.; Gordon, J.: Electrophoretical transfer of proteins from polyacrylamide gels to nitrocellulose sheets: Procedure and some applications. Proc. natn. Acad. Sci. USA *76:*4350–4354 (1979).
10 Laemmli, U. K.: Cleavage of structural proteins during the assembly of the head of bacteriophage T4. Nature, Lond. *227:*680–685 (1970).
11 Bowen, B.; Steinberg, J.; Laemmli, U. K.; Weintraub, H.: The detection of DNA-binding proteins by protein blotting. Nucl. Acids Res. *8:*1–19 (1980).

12 Hunter, W. M.; Greenwood, I. C.: Preparation of Iodine-131-Labeled Human Growth Hormone of High Specific Activity. Nature, Lond. *194:* 495 – 496 (1962).

13 Weissenbach, J.; Chernajovsky, Y.; Jeevi, M.; Shulman, L.; Soreq, H.; Nir, U.; Wallach, D.; Perricaudet, M.; Tiollais, P.; Revel, M.: Two interferon mRNAs in human fibroblasts: In vitro translation and E.coli-cloning studies. Proc. natn. Acad. Sci. USA *77:* 7152 – 7156 (1981).

14 Sagar, A. D.; Pickering, L. A.; Sussman-Berger, V. P.; Stewart, W. E., II; Sehgal, P. B.: Heterogeneity of interferon mRNA species from Sendai-virus-induced human lymphoblastoid (Namalva) cells and Newcastle disease virus-induced murine fibroblastoid (L) cells. Nucl. Acids Res. *9:* 149 – 160 (1980).

Dr. H. K. Hochkeppel, Ges. für Biotechnologische Forschung mbH, Abt. Genetik, Mascheroder Weg 1, D-3300 Braunschweig

Hydrophobicity of Human Interferons

E. Sulkowski and D. V. Goeddel

Roswell Park Memorial Institute, Buffalo, New York and
Genentech, Inc., South San Francisco, California/USA

Introduction

Surface localization of some hydrophobic amino-acid residues [10, 11] gives rise to an *apparent hydrophobicity* of a protein molecule; this hydrophobicity is referred to on occasion as "effective" or "true surface" hydrophobicity. The relative abundance of hydrophobic amino acids, regardless of their localization in a protein molecule, results in an *intrinsic hydrophobicity*.

The propensity of mammalian interferons to enter into hydrophobic interactions has been observed on numerous occasions [16]. However, it still needs to be confirmed with pure preparations of those interferons. It will be also of interest to compare the chromatographic behavior and thus an apparent hydrophobicity of "authentic" interferons produced by mammalian cells with their counterparts produced by "host" cells, bacteria and yeast.

Recently, the amino-acid sequences of several human interferons have been deduced from the nucleotide sequences of their respective cDNA clones [3, 4, 5, 6, 12, 17, 18, 19]. Therefore, it is now possible to calculate and compare the intrinsic hydrophobicities of several human interferons within the interferon family and, in addition, with other proteins as well.

Results

(1) Abundance of Hydrophobic and Aromatic Amino Acids in Human Interferons

Amino-acid compositions of several human interferons are collated in table I. The values for LeIF A, LeIF B, LeIF C, LeIF D, LeIF F, and LeIF H are gleaned from *Goeddel et al.* [6] I, while those for IFN-α1 and IFN-α2 are taken from *Mantei et al.* [12] and *Streuli et al.* [17], respectively. The amino acid composition of IFN-β was reported by *Taniguchi et al.* [19] and independently by others [3, 4].

The content of hydrophobic (L+V+I+M) and aromatic (F+Y+W) amino acids in human interferons is given in table II. There is some variation in the content of those amino acids among α-type (leukocyte) interferons. Nevertheless, it is significantly lower than that of β-type (fibroblast) interferon. Thus, one may register that hydrophobic and aromatic amino-acid residues are more abundant in HuIFN-β than in HuIFN-α.

It is of interest to assess the abundance of hydrophobic and aromatic residues in human interferons vis à vis other unrelated proteins. To this end, the content of hydrophobic and aromatic residues in α-interferons was averaged and expressed as percent. The content of those residues in β-interferon was also expressed as a percent value. The respective values for an *average protein* were taken from Atlas of Protein Sequence and Structure [2]. A perusal at those values, as shown in table III, clearly indicates the relative abundance of hydrophobic and aromatic residues in human interferons by comparison to an average protein.

In order to make this comparison even more succinct, a ratio of the amino acid content in interferons α and β to that in an average protein (AP) was calculated. It is immediately clear that HuIFN-α is enriched in hydrophobic (α/AP = 1.23) and aromatic (α/AP = 1.16) amino acids. This enrichment is particularly conspicuous for HuIFN-β: hydrophobic (β/AP = 1.31) and aromatic (β/AP = 1.60) residues.

(2) Average Hydrophobicity ($H\Phi_{ave}$) of Human Interferons

As a measure of intrinsic hydrophobicity of human interferons we calculated their average hydrophobicities, $H\Phi_{ave}$, a parameter in-

Table I. Amino-acid composition of human interferons

IFN / aa	A	C	D	E	F	G	H	I	K	L	M	N	P	Q	R	S	T	V	W	Y	Total
LeIF A	8	4	8	14	10	5	3	8	11	21	5	4	5	12	9	14	10	7	2	5	165
LeIF B	9	4	12	15	10	2	3	10	10	22	4	4	4	13	10	15	6	7	1	5	166
LeIF C	9	4	8	15	9	5	3	10	7	20	4	6	5	14	13	14	7	7	2	4	166
LeIF D	9	5	11	15	8	3	3	7	8	22	6	6	6	10	12	13	9	7	2	4	166
LeIF F	9	4	7	15	11	5	3	9	10	18	5	6	5	14	10	14	8	8	2	3	166
LeIF H	9	4	7	15	12	2	3	7	9	17	9	9	4	13	12	13	8	7	2	4	166
IFN-α1	10	5	11	15	8	3	3	7	8	22	6	6	6	10	12	13	9	6	2	4	166
IFN-α2	8	4	8	14	10	5	3	8	10	21	5	4	5	12	10	14	10	7	2	5	165
IFN-β	7	3	5	13	9	5	5	11	11	24	4	13	1	10	11	9	7	5	3	10	166

Table II. Content of amino-acid groups in human interferons

HU-IFN	LeIF A	LeIF B	LeIF C	LeIF D	LeIF F	LeIF H	IFN-α1	IFN-α2	IFN-β
A+G	13	11	14	12	14	11	13	13	12
S+T	24	21	21	22	22	21	22	24	16
D+E	22	27	23	26	22	22	26	22	18
D+N+E+Q	38	44	43	42	38	44	42	38	41
K+R+H	23	23	23	23	23	24	23	23	27
L+V+I+M	41	43	41	42	40	40	41	41	44
F+Y+W	17	16	15	14	16	18	14	17	22

Table III. Average percent of amino-acid groups in human interferons and other proteins

aa/Hu-IFN		IFN-α	IFN-β	Average protein (AP)	α/AP	β/AP
Small aliphatic	A+G	7.6	7.2	16.9	0.45	0.43
Hydroxyl	S+T	13.3	9.6	13.1	1.01	0.73
Acidic	D+E	14.4	10.8	11.6	1.24	0.93
Acidic + acid amide	D+N+E+Q	24.8	24.7	19.8	1.25	1.25
Basic	K+R+H	13.9	16.3	13.5	1.03	1.21
Hydrophobic	L+V+I+M	24.8	26.5	20.2	1.23	1.31
Aromatic	F+Y+W	9.6	13.3	8.3	1.16	1.60

Table IV. Average hydrophobicity of human interferons

Hu IFN	α-A		-C	α-D	α-F	α-H	α-1	α-2	β
$H\Phi_{ave}$	1151	1142	1102	1109	1105	1093	1104	1146	1228

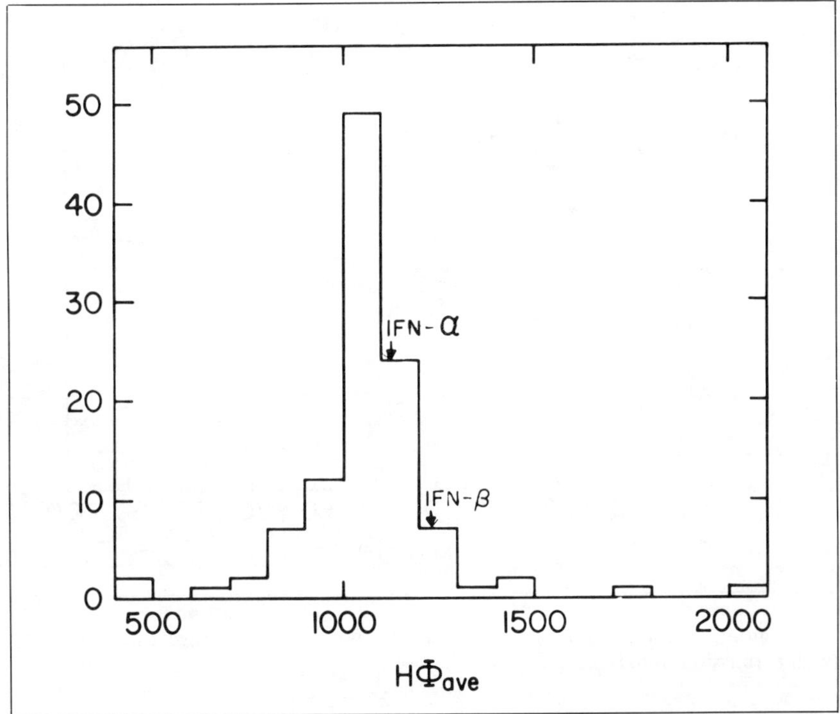

Figure 1. Distribution of average hydrophobicities (with permission from [1]).

troduced by *Bigelow* [1]. The values for individual interferons are given in table IV. The mean value of $H\Phi_{ave}$ for HuIFN-α, 1119, is significantly lower than the value of 1228 for HuIFN-β. Therefore, HuIFN-β is intrinsically more hydrophobic than HuIFN-α.

A comparison of $H\Phi_{ave}$ values for human interferons with those for over 150 unrelated proteins is illustrated in figures 1 and 2. The $H\Phi_{ave}$ values of human interferons are plotted over the original illustrations taken from *Bigelow* [1]. The histogram of the average hydrophobicity values (fig. 1) shows that 50% of the analyzed proteins have $H\Phi_{ave}$ index of 1100. The $H\Phi_{ave}$ value for HuIFN-α, i.e., 1119, falls within 25% portion of proteins having hydrophobic index between 1100 and 1200. The $H\Phi_{ave}$ value for HuIFN-β, i.e., 1228, finds itself within ca. 7% sample of the most hydrophobic proteins.

The diagram of $H\Phi_{ave}$ values plotted against the molecular weights of proteins (fig. 2) shows again that HuIFN-α is somewhat

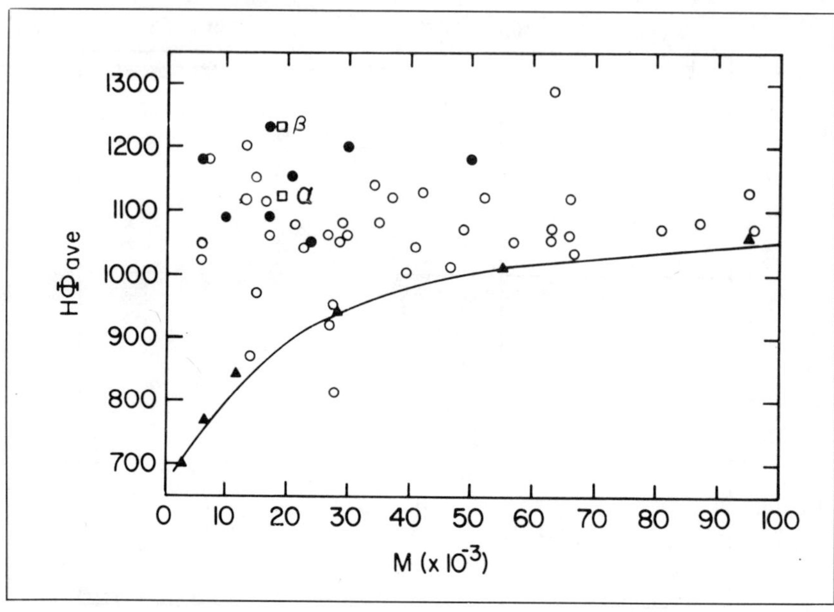

Figure 2. Relationship between molecular weight and average hydrophobicity (with permission from [1]).

more hydrophobic than other proteins of similar size. By contrast, HuIFN-β belongs to the most hydrophobic proteins as sampled by *Bigelow* [1]. Some self-aggregating proteins (closed circles) display high $H\Phi_{ave}$ values (fig. 2). Similarly, the high $H\Phi_{ave}$ value for HuIFN-β may underlie its tendency for the aggregation with other proteins [14].

(3) Aliphatic Index (AI) of Human Interferons

The aliphatic index, AI, defined as the relative volume of a protein occupied by aliphatic side chains (A, V, I, L) was introduced by *Ikai* [7] to assess the thermostability of globular proteins elaborated by thermophilic and mesophilic organisms. The AI calculated for 34 proteins from thermophilic bacteria has x = 92.6 and a standard deviation, s = 10.6. By comparison, AI for proteins (a sample of 208 of non-homologous proteins) derived from mesophilic organisms is x = 78.8 with a standard deviation, s = 14.5.

Table V. Aliphatic index (AI) of human interferons

Hu IFN	LeIF A	LeIF B	LeIF C	LeIF D	LeIF F	LeIF H	IFN-α1	IFN-α2	IFN-β
AI	85.7	82.8	88.1	85.8	82.8	74.1	84.6	85.7	95.2

The AI values calculated for HuIFN-α and HuIFN-β are listed in table V. The x = 83.7 for HuIFN-α is between the values calculated for proteins derived from thermophilic and mesophilic organisms. By comparison, HuIFN-β, although produced by mesophilic organism, has the AI of proteins produced by thermophilic bacteria. Whether thermostability of human interferons can be correlated with their AI values is a matter of conjecture and is best left to the outcome of an experiment. However, it should be noted that the higher AI value for HuIFN-β by comparison to that for HuIFN-α is yet another reflection of their relative intrinsic hydrophobicities.

(4) Distribution of Hydrophobic and Aromatic Amino-Acid Residues along the Interferon Chains

The distribution of hydrophobic (L+V+I+M) and aromatic (F+Y+W) amino acid residues is illustrated in figure 3. The occurrence, if any, of hydrophobic and aromatic residues was ascertained from sequences reported in the literature [6, 12, 17, 19]. Several facets of this distribution deserve some comments: (a) as expected, hydrophobic and aromatic residues are distributed along the whole length of the interferon polypeptide; however, one can identify a small segment in the interferon chain, residues 68 through 77, which is devoid of any hydrophobic and aromatic residues. In effect, this segment "divides" the interferon polypeptide into two large fragments which we will refer to as the "N-fragment" and "C-fragment"; (b) hydrophobic and aromatic residues occur in readily identifiable *clusters,* each about 15 residues long; there are three such clusters, 1-2-3, in the N-fragment and three, 4-5-6, in the C-fragment; (c) the distribution pattern of hydrophobic and aromatic residues is highly conserved within HuIFN-α family; remarkably, there is also a conspicuous similarity in this respect between HuIFN-α and HuIFN-β; (d) the higher content of hydrophobic and aromatic residues in the N- and C-termi-

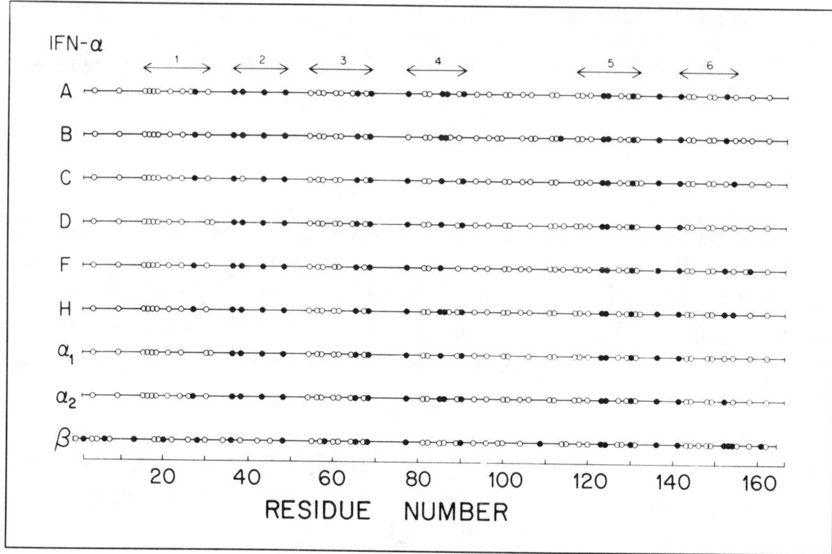

Figure 3. Distribution of hydrophobic + aromatic amino acids.
○ = Hydrophobic amino acids (L + V + I + M).
● = Aromatic amino acids (F + Y + W).

ni of HuIFN-β by comparison to that of HuIFN-α, constitutes the readily discernible difference between β and α human interferons; and (e) phenylalanines are distributed in N- and C-fragments of both HuIFN-α and HuIFN-β; by contrast, tyrosines and tryptophanes are sequestered to the C-fragments in the HuIFN-α family.

(5) Distribution of the Average Hydrophobicity along the Interferon Chains

In order to assess the extent of hydrophobicity along the interferon polypeptide, the local average hydrophobicity was calculated. The interferon polypeptides were arbitrarily divided into consecutive segments of 5 amino-acid residues each. The average hydrophobicity of a 5-residue segment was calculated using hydrophobicity values for amino acids as reported by *Jones* [9]. The results are illustrated in figures 4 and 5 for LeIF A, LeIF B, LeIF C and LeIF D, LeIF F, LeIF H, respectively. A comparison of the distribution of local average hydrophobicities for IFN-α1 and IFN-β is shown in figure 6.

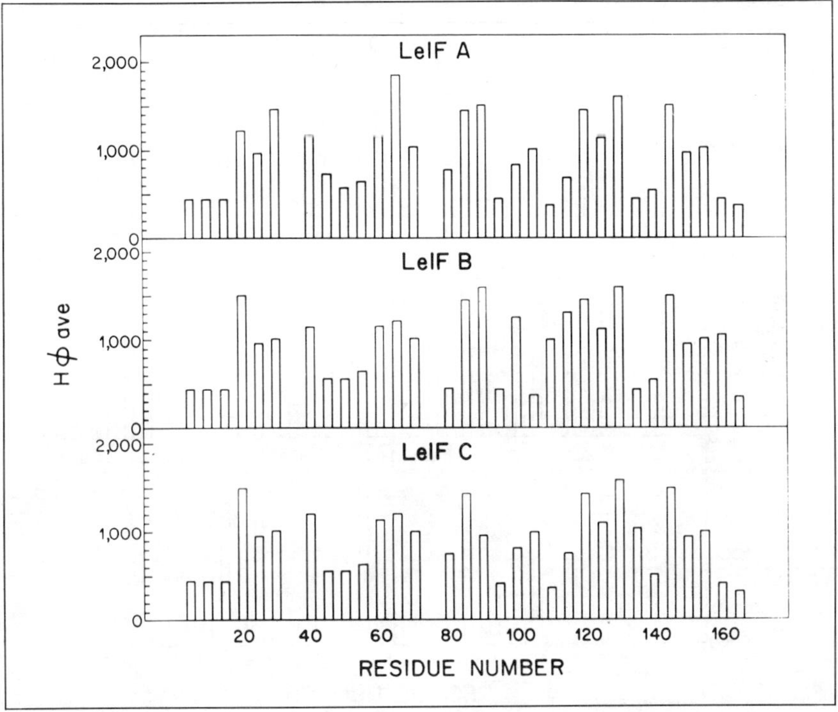

Figure 4. Histogram of hydrophobicity along the interferon chain.

It is clear that the local average hydrophobicity undergoes a considerable fluctuation along the interferon chains. The over-all distribution pattern is, however, common to all members of the HuIFN-α family. Remarkably, there is a striking similarity between HuIFN-α and HuIFN-β in the over-all pattern of the average hydrophobicity.

(6) Hydrophobic Clusters in Human Interferons

The pattern of the distribution of the average hydrophobicity along an interferon polypeptide can be also assessed, and more succinctly so, by the recognition of hydrophobic/aromatic clusters (fig. 3). The values of the average hydrophobicities of 6 such clusters and their adjacent stretches in the interferon chains have been calculated for IFN-α1 and IFN-β. The results are illustrated in figure 7.

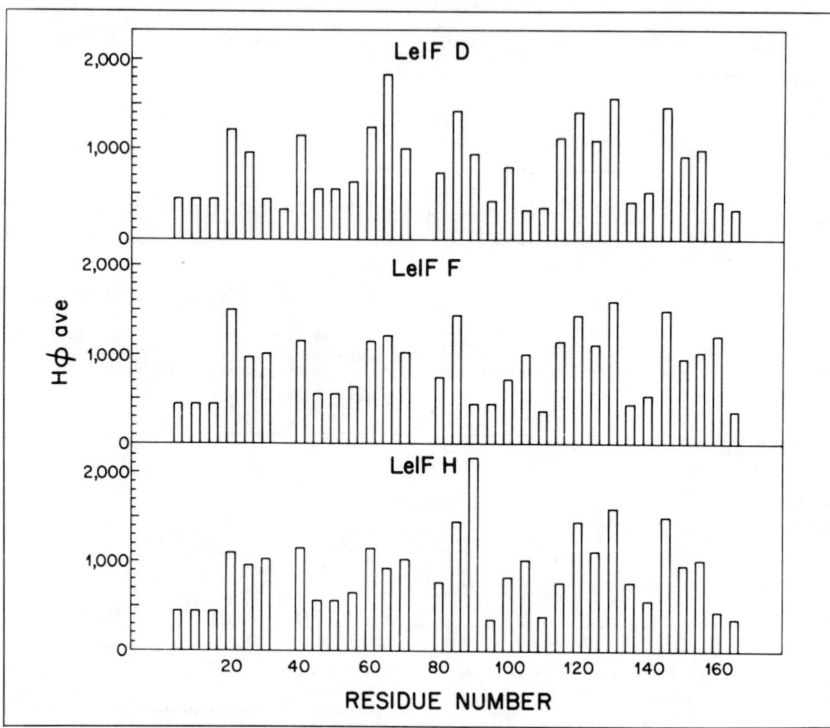

Figure 5. Histogram of hydrophobicity along the interferon chain.

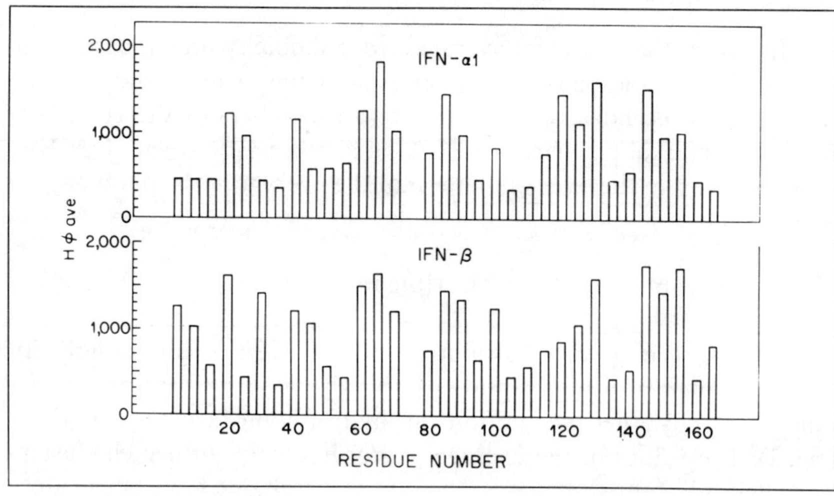

Figure 6. Histogram of hydrophobicity along the interferon chain.

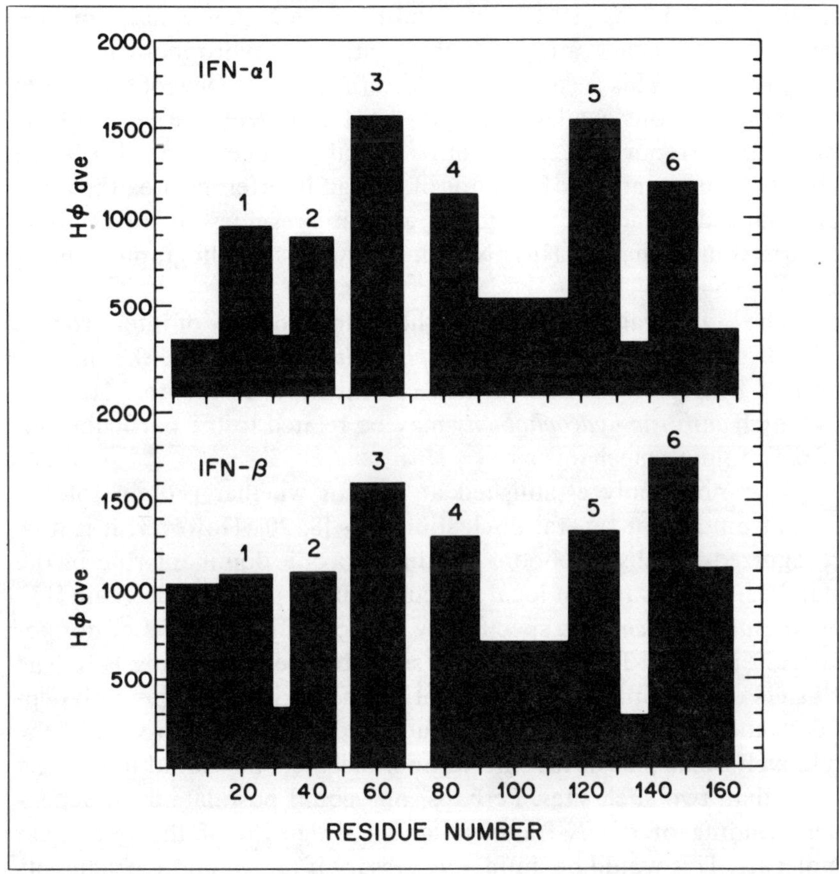

Figure 7. **Histogram of hydrophobicity distribution along the interferon chain.**

The similarity of IFN-α1 and IFN-β, in terms of the distribution of the average hydrophobicities along their chains, is quite compelling. It is also clear that the only conspicuous difference between the two occurs at their N- and C-termini.

Discussion

The hydrophobic properties of human interferons were initially unraveled by the chromatography on a variety of hydrophobic ligands. On the basis of their chromatographic behavior, it was postulated previously that HuIFN-β should have a higher content of aromatic amino acids and a higher intrinsic hydrophobicity than HuIFN-α [16]. This seems to be indeed the case, in view of the amino acid compositions available now [6, 12, 17, 19] and as a result of the calculations reported here. Another specific expectation, also based on the chromatographic behavior of human interferons, i.e., the more pronounced surface localization of aromatic residues on HuIFN-β by comparison to that on HuIFN-α, must await crystallographic analysis.

The biological significance of the hydrophobicity of interferons is still obscure. Their *apparent hydrophobicity* may underlie the interaction of interferon molecules with cell-membrane receptors [15, 16]. The high *intrinsic hydrophobicity* may be related to the particularities of their folding mechanisms.

It is not firmly established at present whether protein folding starts from one or several nucleation sites [8, 20]. However, it is now recognized that hydrophobic bonding plays a dominant role in the stabilization of transient local structures in the polypeptide chain [13]. *Matheson* and *Scheraga* specifically proposed that pockets of nonpolar residues may form nucleation sites for protein folding [13]. The clusters of hydrophobic and aromatic residues in interferon polypeptide could conceivably constitute such nucleation sites. In view of the relatively small size of the interferon molecule, one should not expect more than two such sites. Perhaps, one could postulate an independent folding of the N-fragment and C-fragment of the interferon molecule. This would be, in fact, necessary if the N- and C-fragments were to form continuous domains [20]. An additional and maybe the most important question to ask is whether a particular fragment of the interferon molecule can assume a native-like tertiary conformation and perhaps display some biological activity. In view of the potential of both recombinant-DNA technology and solid-phase synthesis, these may not be premature questions.

References

1 Bigelow, C. C.: On the average hydrophobicity of proteins and the relation between it and protein structure. J. theoret. Biol. *16:* 187–211 (1967).

2 Dayhoff, M. O.; Hunt, L. T.; Hurst-Calderone, S.: Composition of proteins. In Atlas of Protein Sequence and Structure *5:* suppl. 3, p. 363 (1978).

3 Derynck, R.; Content, J.; DeClercq, E.; Volckaert, G.; Tavernier, J.; Devos, R.; Fiers, W.: Isolation and structure of a human fibroblast interferon gene. Nature *285:* 542–546 (1980).

4 Goeddel, D. V.; Shepard, H. M.; Yeverton, E.; Leung, D.; Crea, R.: Synthesis of human fibroblast interferon by E. coli. Nucl. Acids Res. *8:* 4057–4074 (1980).

5 Goeddel, D. V.; Yelverton, E.; Ullrich, A.; Heyneker, H. L.; Miozzari, G.; Holmes, W.; Seeburg, P. H.; Dull, T.; May, L.; Stebbing, N.; Crea, R.; Maeda, S.; McCandliss, R.; Sloma, A.; Tabor, J. M.; Gross, M.; Familetti, P. C.; Pestka, S.: Human leukocyte interferon produced by E. coli is biologically active. Nature *287:* 411–416 (1980).

6 Goeddel, D. V.; Leung, D. W.; Dull, T. J.; Gross, M.; Lawn, R. M.; McCandliss, R.; Seeburg, P. H.; Ullrich, A.; Yelverton, E.; Gray, P. W.: The structure of eight distinct cloned human leukocyte interferon cDNAs. Nature *290:* 20–26 (1981).

7 Ikai, A.: Thermostability and aliphatic index of globular proteins. J. Biochem. Tokyo *88:* 1895–1898 (1980).

8 Johanson, K. O.; Wetlaufer, D. B.; Reed, R. G.; Peters, T., Jr.: Refolding of bovine serum albumin and its proteolytic fragments. J. biol. Chem. *256:* 445–450 (1981).

9 Jones, D. D.: Amino-acid properties and side-chain orientation in proteins: A cross correlation approach. J. theor. Biol. *50:* 167–183 (1975).

10 Klotz, I. M.: Comparison of molecular structures of proteins: Helix content; Distribution of apolar residues. Archs. Biochem. Biophys. *138:* 704–706 (1970).

11 Lee, B.; Richards, F. M.: The interpretation of protein structures: Estimation of static accessibility. J. mol. Biol. *55:* 379–400 (1971).

12 Mantei, N.; Schwarzstein, M.; Streuli, M.; Panem, S.; Nagata, S.; Weissmann, C.: The nucleotide sequence of a cloned human leukocyte interferon cDNA. Gene *10:* 1–10 (1980).

13 Matheson, R. R.; Scheraga, H. A.: A method for predicting nucleation sites for protein folding based on hydrophobic contacts. Macromolecules *11:* 819–828 (1978).

14 Reynolds, F. H.; Pitha, P. M.: Molecular weight study of human fibroblast interferon. Biochem. biophys. Res. Commun. *65:* 107–112 (1975).

15 Sulkowski, E.; Davey, M. W.; Carter, W. A.: Interaction of human interferons with immobilized hydrophobic amino acids and dipeptides. J. biol. Chem. *251:* 5381–5385 (1976).

16 Sulkowski, E.; Vastola, K.; Le, H. V.: Hydrophobic properties of interferons. Ann. N. Y. Acad. Sci. *350:* 339–346 (1980).

17 Streuli, M.; Nagata, S.; Weissmann, C.: At least three human type α interferons: Structure of α2. Science *209:* 1343–1347 (1980).

18 Taniguchi, T.; Mantei, N.; Schwarzstein, M.; Nagata, S.; Muramatsu, M.; Weissmann, C.: Human leukocyte and fibroblast interferons are structurally related. Nature *285:* 547–549 (1980).

19 Taniguchi, T.; Ohno, S.; Fujii-Kuriyama, Y.; Muramatsu, M.: The nucleotide sequence of human fibroblast interferon cDNA. Gene *10:* 11–15 (1980).

20 Wetlaufer, D. B.: Nucleation, rapid folding, and globular intrachain regions in proteins. Proc. natn. Acad. Sci. USA *70:* 697–701 (1973).

Eugene Sulkowski, PhD, Roswell Park Memorial Institute, 666 Elm Street, USA-Buffalo, NY 14263

Biological Activities of Pure HuIFN-α Species

Kurt Berg, Marianne Hokland, Iver Heron

Institute of Medical Microbiology, University of Aarhus, Denmark

Introduction

During the last five years it has become evident that HuIFN-α, besides its antiviral activity, is able to influence a broad variety of cellular functions [12, 15] especially on cells belonging to the white blood cell system [7 – 12]. The NK system has in particular drawn considerable interest, although it might be argued that it is "only" an in vitro technique, the clinical relevance of which has not yet been convincingly demonstrated [*Strander,* 1981, personal communication]. Most of the observations were originally done by means of crude or partially purified interferon preparations which are known to be contaminated with a variety of lymphokines [14]. Thus, it was difficult to conclude if the observed effects were due to impurities present in the interferon preparations or to the interferon molecule itself. Although many "indirect" experiments were performed as controls (example: no effect was seen with mock interferon preparations, etc.), the ultimate answer to the question, if all the biological activities ascribed to the interferon molecules are harbored exclusively in the interferon molecules themselves, implies the use of pure HuIFN-α species (pure by SDS-PAGE).

Very recently, our group [4] has reported on the purification of HuIFN-α by combining gelfiltration with different ligand chromatographies (incl. antibody-affinity chromatography). The purified preparations were examined in SDS-PAGE and it was demonstrated that only interferon proteins were present [4].

In the following four (i–iv) different non-viral properties were checked by means of pure HuIFN-α species: (i) antiproliferative effect; (ii) potentiation of the NK-system; (iii) cytotoxic T-cell assay, and (iv) the expression of β_2-microglobulin on lymphocytes. Furthermore, antigenic characterization of 2 of the major species of HuIFN-α (18,000 and 22,000) prompted the production of antibodies which turned out to be highly useful for purification of HuIFN-α. Finally, the problem of the number of species of HuIFN-α present in human leukocyte interferon were examined in a modified SDS-PAGE.

Results and Discussion

Crude human leukocyte (generously provided by K. Osther, Alfred Benzon A/S, Copenhagen) was purified according to the previously published procedures involving gelfiltration, ligand- and antibody-affinity chromatographies yielding 50% recovery together with a specific activity of about $10^8 - 10^9$ units/mg proteins [4]. This material was divided into two aliquots and examined in an SDS-PAGE (25 cm long slab 8 – 22% acrylamide gradient gel) simultaneously for proteins and biological activities. Several protein bands were demonstrated subsequent to staining in Coomassie Blue (for technical details see [1 – 4]). As can be seen from figure 1 (lower part) all the proteins are located at the exact same positions as the biological activities eluted from the unstained part of the gel. Thus it can be concluded that all the proteins, seen as stained bands in the SDS-PAGE, are interferon proteins [4]. The eluted interferon (from the unstained part of the gel) served as pure interferon proteins. They were used in the following assays:

(1) Inhibition of growth of the Daudi-cells, measured by the inhibition of the thymidine-uptake.
(2) Stimulation of natural-killer cell (NK) activity.
(3) Enhanced expression on lymphocytes of HLA antigens.
(4) Augmented alloreactive T-killer cell generation in vitro.

As can be seen in figure 1 (lower part) the antiviral activity (full line) and the relative growth inhibition (broken line, upper part of fig. 1) follow each other very closely. Even the small interferon peak at 19,500 can also be detected, provided another dilution range is chosen (not shown; for more technical information, see [3]). Thus from

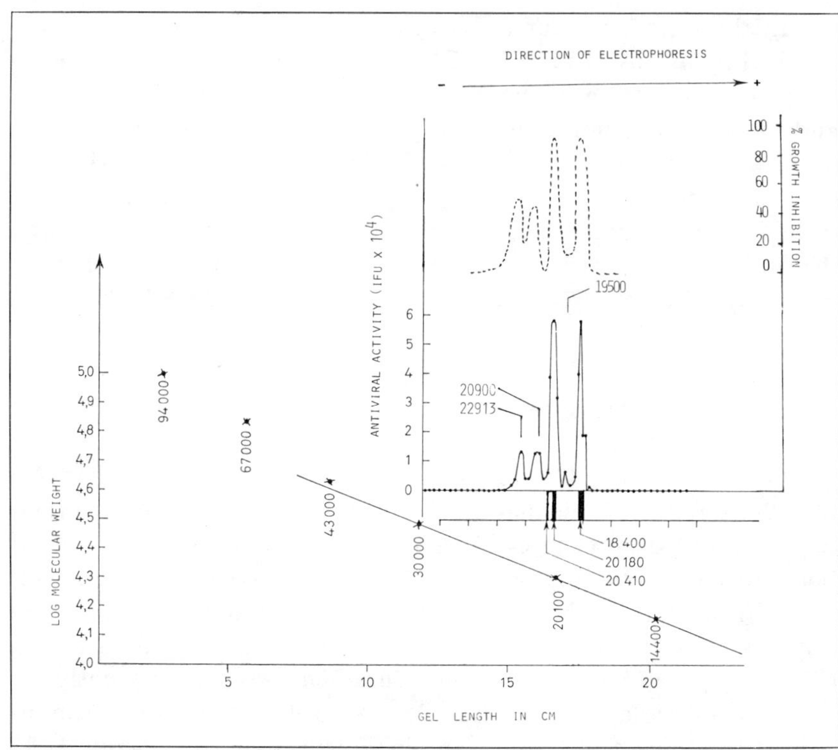

Figure 1. Separation of purified human leukocyte interferon into different species by SDS-PAGE. About 2×10^6 IFU of purified HuIFN-α were divided into two portions which were loaded into two separate slots. After electrophoresis, one of the interferon-containing gel strips was cut out, divided into 1 mm pieces, eluted and titrated for antiviral activity (●——●). The remaining part of the gel was stained, destained, and dried, and the locations of the protein bands were plotted. The upper curve shows the anticellular activity (– – –) of the interferon fractions, tested at a dilution of 1:1000, in terms of inhibition of thymidine uptake, expressed as a percentage of that in control cultures. ×, Mol. wt.

the data presented in figure 1 one would be tempted to favor the hypothesis that the anticellular activity in a leukocyte interferon preparation is harbored only in the interferon molecules [13]. This statement needs to be evaluated more thoroughly before a final conclusion can be made due to the following findings: the species of the pure interferon (fig. 1) were compared with a partially purified human leukocyte interferon preparation (PIF) as currently used in the clinics (specific activity was 1×10^6 units/mg protein) in the Daudi-cell system. Both preparations were found equal, unit for unit, regarding inhibition of growth of the Daudi-cells. However, replacing the Daudi-cells with U-cells yielded a significant difference. The PIF-preparations is about 10 times more effective, unit for unit, compared to the pure interferon species. This seems to indicate that 90% of the anticellular activity present in a PIF-preparation is not due exclusively to the interferon proteins. Rather, there might be some "lymphokines" present in the PIF which exert part of the major anticellular activity. The reason for not finding this "extra" activity in the Daudi-system could be due to differences in receptors. Thus the U-cells are not able to recognize these "lymphokines". This in a way supports the findings of *Dahl* [5, 6].

One might also argue that the SDS (0.1%), which is unavoidable for the final separation of the HuIFN-α species, would influence the assay system in such a manner that the anticellular activity of IFN in some systems would become less pronounced. Alternatively, one could also envision that part(s) of the native interferon molecule is destroyed by the SDS-treatment. Further analyses are needed before any final conclusions can be made. The same problem regarding the efficiency of PIF vs. the pure HuIFN-α species (stabilized with SDS), unit for unit, might also apply to other non-viral systems.

The species of HuIFN-α (18,000, 20,000, and 22,000 (fig. 2)) were assessed for regulatory functions in the NK-system, the HLA-system, and the T-cell system.

The results from one representative experiment in the NK-system is shown in figure 2 (upper part). The lymphoblastoid T-cell line ALL-1301 was used as target cell. Peripheral blood lymphocytes from healthy laboratory personnel were incubated separately in tubes at 1×10^6 per ml in TC199 10% FCS for 1 h at 37°C together with the 3 interferon species. SDS-buffers in proper dilutions and eluted gel fractions containing no interferon activity as well as normal medium served as controls for "base-line" NK-activity. PIF, diluted to contain similar numbers of antiviral units per ml as the 3 species, was used as "positive control". Lymphocytes were then washed twice and added to ^{51}Cr-labeled target cells at a ratio 25:1. After 4 h of incubation ^{51}Cr release was estimated.

From figure 2 it will be seen that all of the 3 IFN species examined contain NK-boosting activity, as does PIF [7, 10, 12].

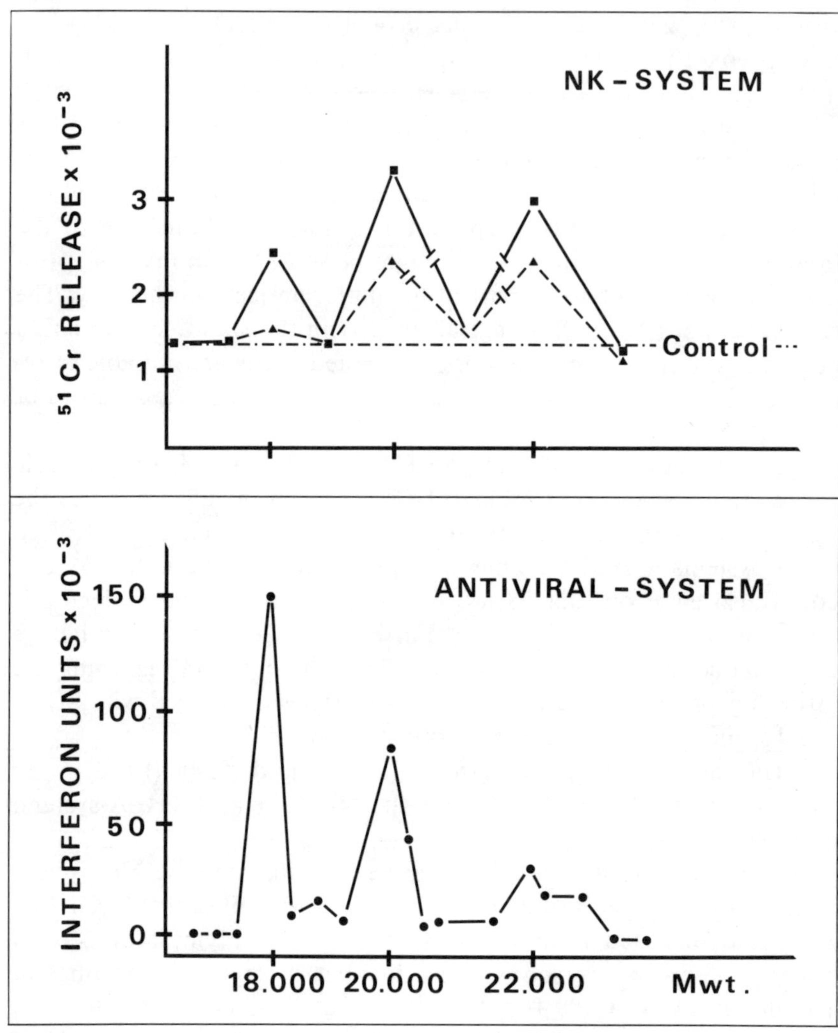

Figure 2. The stimulation of the natural-killer cells (NK) by the 3 HuIFN-α species (18,000, 20,000, and 22,000) using 50 units of IFN (▲) or 500 units of IFN per ml (■). For further details, see the text.

The 18,000-fraction has been found to express somewhat less activity per antiviral unit than the 20,000- and 22,000-MW fractions as shown also in figure 2. Whether this reflects significant differences between the native species or only minor differences in a possible SDS-denaturation remains to be seen (see later in this section).

Normal lymphocytes, kept overnight in culture in medium 10% human serum, were used for measurement of IFN-induced changes in expression of major histocompatibility antigens (MHC) on the membrane. Following the incubation in the presence of the various interferon preparations and appropriate controls, the quantitation of MHC was mostly done after staining with FITC-conjugated rabbit antihuman β_2-microglobulin antibodies (Dako-Patts, Copenhagen). Cells were then assessed for fluorescence in a FACS II and the mean relative fluorescence intensity per cell was calculated. The same 3 HuIFN-α species possessed also the capacity to induce a similar increase in the fluorescence intensity when compared unit for unit, confirming the previous findings of *Heron et al.* [11].

In mixed lymphocyte reactions (MLR) added IFN has previously been found to generate higher cell-mediated lympholysis (CML) potential than parallel control of MLR [8, 9, 12]. The same 3 HuIFN-α species were tested in this system at 500 antiviral units per ml at the same concentration which was found optimal for PIF [8, 9]. Each of the species proved to possess activity in this system although the 18,000-species was again somewhat inferior to that of the 2 others, unit for unit.

To summarize the above experiments all 3 species of HuIFN-α yielded the same effects as described with partially purified interferon preparations, although there appears to be some quantitative differences regarding the efficacy between the individual species unit for unit.

It was shown by *Berg and Heron* [4] that most of the HuIFN-α species can withstand the staining (Coomassie Blue) and destaining treatment, although some loss of biological activity occurred (the antigenic properties remained remarkably stable). Thus it is possible to obtain pure (stained) separated interferon proteins (in acrylamide) by performing an SDS-PAGE, subsequent to staining, destaining, and gelcutting. Therefore, a minor part of the gel was minced (by a teflon rod) before elution and titration for interferon activity. The remainder part was used as is and injected directly into a rabbit (incl. Freund's adjuvants, biweekly) using a total amount of $1-2 \times 10^6$ units (input to the SDS-PAGE).

Antibodies against the 18,000- and 22,000-species were developed after 4 months with relatively low titers (3000 and 100 respectively). It was shown that these antibodies were able to neutralize both interferon species completely in an identical manner. Thus, based on rabbit anti-interferon sera, the 2 major species appear antigenically identical. Analogous findings were seen with the 20,000-species.

The IgG-fractions from the antisera against the 18,000- and 20,000-species were isolated after protein-A chromatography, and 2 anti-interferon columns were constructed according to previous reports [1 – 4]. Both columns were able, in one step, to purify gelfiltered (crude) interferon to the same level as depicted in figure 1 (lower part). However, it was noticed that eluates, obtained from the antibody column made against the 20,000-species, contained less proteins at the 18,000-location in the subsequent SDS-PAGE than eluates obtained from the antibody column directed against the 18,000-species.

This prompted a reinvestigation of the purified interferon preparation (fig. 1). Modifying the SDS-PAGE system by changing the acrylamide-gel gradient (see legend to fig. 3) yielded a separating system which was able to distinguish among the interferon species even further (fig. 3) compared to the previous technique ([4] and fig. 1). As can be seen in figure 3, 13 different species of HuIFN-α were separated and characterized. The apparent molecular weights have decreased with 1000 – 1500 compared to the molecular markers for reasons not clearly understood. Thus, the original 18,000-band (fig. 1) could be resolved further into 4 separate interferon peaks (slice 1 – 4, fig. 3) of which the major protein (containing 40% of the total protein content of all 13 species as judged by the intensity of the stain) is located at 16,600 (slice 1, fig. 3). One might expect the highest interferon content to be located in the fraction containing the highest amount of proteins. Otherwise, one could argue that the major protein, which was found in gel slice 1, is not an interferon protein at all.

Before embarking on a conclusion it should also be noted that the profile in figure 1 is derived from an unstained gel ("native" SDS interferon), whereas the profile in figure 3 stems from a stained and destained SDS-PAGE. Therefore, a certain inactivation of the interferon might have occurred. However, *Berg* and *Heron* [4] showed that only a minor loss occurred at the 18,000-location under such regimen compared to the 20,000-species. Thus it is likely that slice 1 contains almost no interferon activity in the native stage in contrast to gel slices 2 – 4 representing the species containing the major part of the biological activity originally ascribed to the 18,000-species (fig. 1). It

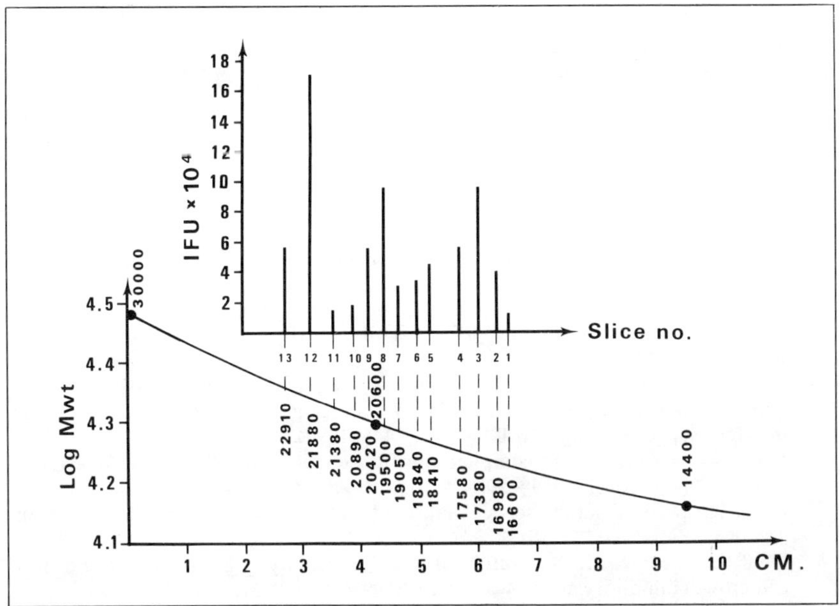

Figure 3. 3×10^6 units of purified HuIFN-α were loaded in one slot to a 20 cm long polyacrylamide-gel slab (0.75 mm thick) including a 10 cm stacking gel (3%). The first 10 cm consisted of a 12–25% acrylamide gradient and the remainder 10 cm consisted of 25% acrylamide. After electrophoresis, the gel was stained for 15 min and destained for 20 min and washed twice with distilled water. The precise locations of 13 separated protein bands were noted (some of which were rather faint). Each band was cut out of the gel, minced with a teflon rod and eluted separately in 0.5 ml 0.01% SDS-solution, and titrated for IFN-activity. Molecular markers (14,400, 20,600, and 30,000) were included in a parallel gel-slot (●).

turned out, however, that slice 1 had an extremely high antiviral activity in the bovine system [15], thus ruling out the possibility that the proteins in slice 1 should be a non-interferon protein (further experiments are in progress).

In summary, HuIFN-α seems to consist of at least 13 different species, as judged by SDS-PAGE, of which one, representing 40% of the total protein, has almost no activity in the human system, but a high activity in the bovine system. Further experiments are needed to disclose which properties and what roles this species might play in the human interferon system, if any.

Acknowledgments

The authors are indebted to the excellent technical assistance provided by *K. Vestergård, K. Durup,* and *I. Sørensen.* This investigation was supported by the Danish Cancer Society.

References

1 Berg, K.: Sequential antibody-affinity chromatography of human leukocyte interferon. Scand. J. Immunol. *6:* 77 – 86 (1977).
2 Berg, K.; Heron, I.; Hamilton, R.: Purification of human interferons by antibody-affinity chromatography, using highly absorbed anti-interferon. Scand. J. Immunol. *8:* 429 – 436 (1978).
3 Berg, K.; Heron, I.: SDS-polyacrylamide gel electrophoresis of purified human leukocyte interferon and the antiviral and anticellular activities of the different interferon species. J. gen. Virol. *50:* 441 – 446 (1980).
4 Berg, K.; Heron, I.: The complete purification of human leukocyte interferon. Scand. J. Immunol. *11:* 489 – 502 (1980).
5 Dahl, H.: Differentiation between antiviral and anticellular effects of interferon. Tex. Rep. Biol. Med. *35:* 381 – 387 (1977).
6 Dahl, H.; Degree, M.: Separation of antiviral activity of human interferon from cell growth inhibitory effect. Nature *257:* 799 – 801 (1975).
7 Herberman, R. R.; Ortaldo, J. R.; Bounard, G. D.: Augmentation by interferon of human natural and antibody-dependent cell-mediated cytotoxicity. Nature *277:* 221 – 223 (1979).
8 Heron, I.; Berg, K.; Cantell, K.: Regulatory effect of interferon on T-cells in vitro. J. Immun. *117:* 1370 – 1373 (1976).
9 Heron, I.; Berg, K.: Human leukocyte interferon: Analysis of effect on MLC and effector cell generation. Scand. J. Immunol. *9:* 517–526 (1979).
10 Heron, I.; Hokland, M.; Møller-Larsen, A.; Berg, K.: The effect of interferon on lymphocyte-mediated effector cell functions: Selective enhancement of natural-killer cells. Cell. Immunol. *42:* 183 – 187 (1979).
11 Heron, I.; Hokland, M.; Berg, K.: Enhanced expression of β_2-microglobulin and HLA-antigens on human lymphoid cells by interferon. Proc. natn. Acad. Sci. USA *75:* 6215 – 6219 (1978).
12 Heron, I.; Hokland, M.; Hokland, P.; Berg, K.: Effects of interferon on human lymphoid cells and their functions. Ann. N. Y. Acad. Sci. *350:* 112–120 (1980).
13 Stewart, W. E., II Gresser, I.; Tovey, M.; Bander, M.; LeGoff, S.: Identification of the cell-multiplication-inhibitory factors in interferon preparations as interferons. Nature *262:* 300–302 (1976).
14 Stewart, W. E., II: The Interferon System (Springer Verlag, Berlin 1979).
15 Stewart, W. E., II: Varied biological effects of interferon. Interferon *1:* 29 – 46 (1979).

Prof. Dr. Kurt Berg, Institute of Medical Microbiology, Bartholin Building, University of Aarhus, DK-8000 Aarhus C

Characterization of Human (β) Fibroblast Interferon

E. Knight, Jr.[1], *D. C. Blomstrom*[1], *M. W. Hunkapiller*[2]

[1] Central Research and Development Department, E. I. du Pont de Nemours & Co., Wilmington, Delaware, USA
[2] Biology Division, California Institute of Technology, Pasadena, California, USA

Introduction

The characterization of interferons produced by animal cells is essential in order (1) to understand the molecular mechanisms involved in the phenomena induced by interferons and (2) to maximize the clinical utility of the interferons. Our goal has been to study the chemical properties of pure human fibroblast (β) interferon including the determination of its amino-acid sequence.

Methods and Results

Human fibroblast (β) interferon is produced from human diploid fibroblast (FS4-cells) on induction by poly I:C [1, 2]. A 2-step purification procedure has been developed that yields fibroblast interferon of greater than 95% purity [3]. Both steps in the purification involve chromatography on agarose containing covalently bound Cibacron Blue (Blue Sepharose, Pharmacia, Inc.). Crude interferon is passed through a large column of Blue Sepharose under conditions whereby the interferon binds to the column but most of the contaminating proteins do not. The interferon is then eluted from the column with a buffer containing 50% ethylene glycol. To concentrate the interferon and obtain a purity of greater than 95%, it is fractionated again on Blue Sepharose but on a much smaller column. After extensive washing of the column the interferon is eluted with ethylene glycol. The elution of the interferon from the large and small columns is shown

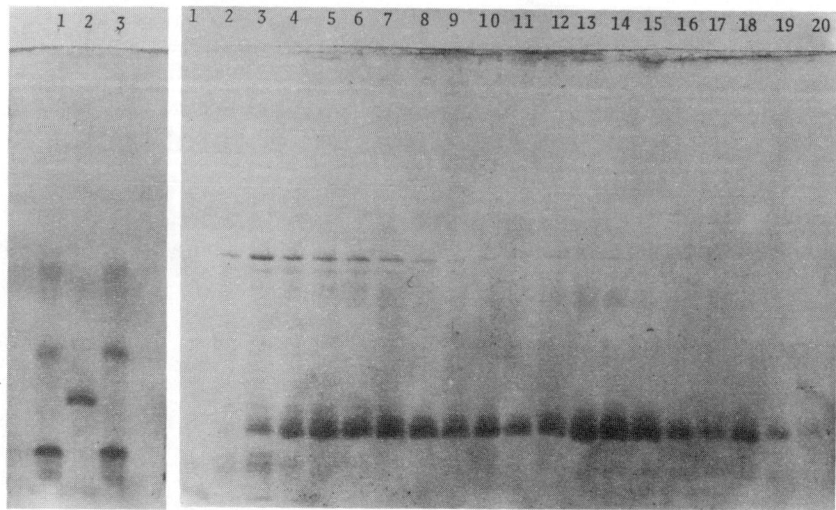

Figure 1. Chromatography of human fibroblast interferon on Blue Sepharose. (a) Large column, fractions 15–23 pooled. (b) Small column, fractions 22–23 pooled.

Figure 2. Analysis by SDS-polyacrylamide gel electrophoresis of fractions from small Blue Sepharose column. Tracks 2–20 are 0.5 ml of fraction 4, 6, 8– – – –40 respectively.

in figure 1. The yield of interferon and final specific activity obtained by the aforementioned procedure are shown in table I. Yields of biological activity have ranged from 20% to 40%. The purification factor from the crude interferon is 2900-fold.

When the interferon fractions, obtained from the second Blue Sepharose column, are analyzed by electrophoresis on a SDS-polyacrylamide gel, one predominant band is detected after staining with Coomassie Blue (fig. 2). When fractions 8–20 are pooled and analyzed by electrophoresis only one band is detected (fig. 3). The interferon activity comigrates with this band and has an estimated molecular weight of 20,000.

The interferon, purified by the procedure shown in table I and analyzed by electrophoresis as shown in figures 1 and 2, has been used for amino-acid sequencing. The N-terminal amino-acid sequence for fibroblast interferon has been reported [4]. The N-terminal amino-acid sequence of the interferon, purified by the procedure shown in table I, is the same as that obtained by another purification procedure and reported previously [4]. There was the only N-terminal

Table I. Purification of human fibroblast interferon

Fraction	Volume ml	Ref. unit interferon	Protein mg	Specific activity	% Rec.
Crude	10,000	85×10^6	500	1.7×10^5	100
1st Blue Sepharose col. 1 m NaCl, 50% E. G.	160	68×10^6	0.6	1×10^8	80
2nd Blue Sepharose col. 2 m NaCl, 40% E. G.	10	30×10^6	0.06	5×10^8	35

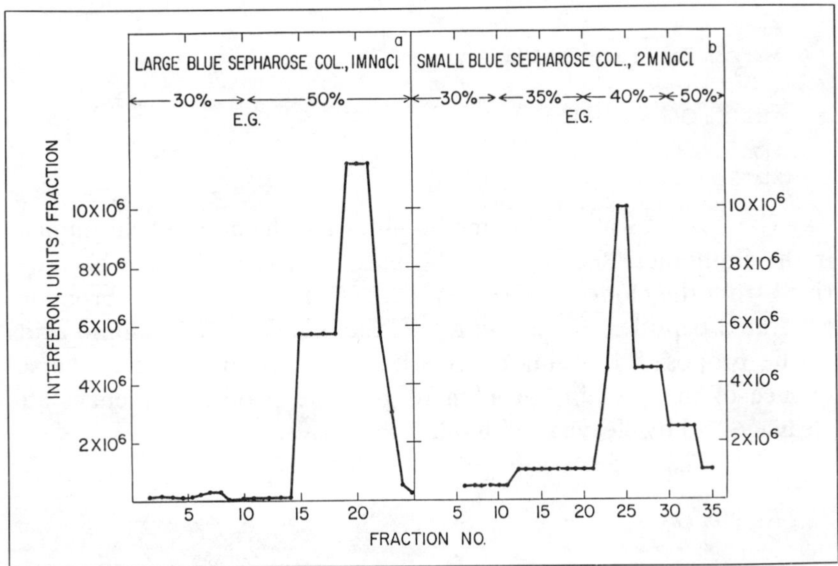

Figure 3. Analysis by SDS-polyacrylamide electrophoresis of pooled small Blue Sepharose column fractions.

sequence observed indicating that the interferon is at least 95% pure. This degree of purity is acceptable for chemical characterization of the interferon. Furthermore, the N-terminal sequence of the fibroblast interferon is identical to that obtained by *Taniguchi et al.* [5] after cloning in *E. coli* and sequencing the presumed fibroblast interferon structural gene.

To complete the amino-acid sequence of the interferon protein, it is necessary to produce peptides with either chemicals or proteolytic enzymes. We have chosen cyanogen bromide for it should produce only a small number of peptides since it cleaves only at methionine residues. Peptides generated by cleavage with cyanogen bromide were separated by electrophoresis in SDS-polyacrylamide gel. The N-terminal sequences of the peptides were determined by a microsequencing technique [6]. The N-terminal sequence and the sequences of internal peptides generated by cyanogen bromide are shown as follows:

N Terminus
1
Met Ser Tyr Asn Leu Leu Gly Phe Leu Gln Arg Ser Ser Asn

Phe Gln Cys Gln Lys Leu Leu

36
Met Asn Phe Asp Ile Pro Glu

62
Met Leu Gln Asn Ile Phe

117
Met Ser Ser Leu.

The numbers above the methionines are the amino-acid number in the amino-acid sequence of fibroblast interferon that has been derived from the cloned cDNA sequence [5]. From cyanogen-bromide-generated peptides we have obtained the sequence of 38 amino acids of the proposed 166 amino acids [5]. In order to complete the sequence of the protein, we plan to generate peptides by enzymatic cleavage and by cleavage with other chemicals.

References

1 Havell, E. A.; Vilcek, J.: Production of High-Titered Interferons in Cultures of Human Diploid Cells. Antimicrob. Agents Chemother. *2:* 476–484 (1972).

2 Knight, E., Jr.: Interferon: Purification and Initial Characterization from Human Diploid Cells. Proc. natn. Acad. Sci. USA *73:* 520–523 (1976).

3 Knight, E., Jr.; Fahey, D.: Human Fibroblast Interferon: An Improved Purification. J. biol. Chem. *256:* 3609–3611 (1981).

4 Knight, E., Jr.; Hunkapiller, M. W.; Korant, B. D.; Hardy, R. W. F.; Hood, L. E.: Human Fibroblast Interferon: Amino Acid Analysis and Amino Terminal Amino Acid Sequence. Science *207:* 525–526 (1980).

5 Taniguchi, T.; Ohno, S.; Fujii-Kuriyama, Y.; Muramatsu, M.: The Nucleotide Sequenator of Human Fibroblast Interferon cDNA. Gene *10:* 11–15 (1980).

6 Hunkapiller, M. W.; Hood, L. E.: New Protein Sequenator with Increased Sensitivity. Science *207:* 523–525 (1980).

Prof. Dr. E. Knight, Jr., Central Research & Development Dep., Experimental Station, Bldg. 328, E. I. du Pont de Nemours & Co., USA-Wilmington, Delaware 19 898

Studies with Lymphoblastoid Interferon

N. B. Finter, G. Allen, G. D. Ball, K. H. Fantes, M. Johnston, T. Priestman

Wellcome Research Laboratories, Langley Court, Beckenham, Kent, England

Nearly all the interferon so far used in patients has been made from human white blood ("buffy coat") cells by *Strander* and *Cantell's* procedure described in 1966 [1]. Most interferon has been made in Finland, and although the product, PIF, is less than 1% pure, it has proved to be perfectly acceptable for clinical use. Nevertheless, cells derived from individual units of human blood are not an ideal source for the manufacture of interferon, and could not provide sufficient amounts to enable the wide-spread use of interferon in routine clinical practice. From both points of view, it would be preferable to make interferon from some cell which can be grown on a large scale. Therefore, in 1974, encouraged by the results already obtained with Finnish leukocyte interferon, and since there seemed to be no realistic alternative, we decided to explore the production of interferon from human transformed cells. At that time, it was generally held that a product for use in man should not be made from such cells, because it was feared that this might lead to its contamination with some carcinogenic agent. In fact, no such agent has ever been identified in human transformed cells. We decided that it was reasonable to use them as a source of interferon for clinical use, provided that the final product was purified sufficiently and by a process likely to render it safe.

We started to test a number of human transformed cell lines, but, impressed by the data of *Strander, Mogensen* and *Cantell* [2], we decided to concentrate on human lymphoblastoid cells. After screening some 150 lines [3], we selected one line termed Namalwa, which had already been identified as a high interferon yielder [2], for further study.

We have devised systems for growing Namalwa cells on a considerable scale, and making interferon from them. Our initial pilot plant was based on a cell-culture tank of 1,000 l capacity, from which, at intervals, 600 l of cell suspension were withdrawn and stimulated with Sendai virus to form interferon. After separation of the cells, the crude interferon was purified by a multi-stage procedure which also served to "decontaminate" it, as shown by the destruction or elimination of various marker substances deliberately added to experimental batches of crude interferon. These markers included many different viruses, nucleic acids, mycoplasmas, bacteria, bacterial endotoxin, and even scrapie agent (a slow virus infection of mice, which is extremely resistant to inactivation by chemical or physical means). More details about such tests have been given elsewhere [4]. We are now operating an industrial-scale production and purification plant which routinely provides a mixture of at least 8 different leukocyte-type interferons [5, 6] in high purity (specific activity usually not less than 10^8 International Units per mg total protein). We have also developed an objective physico-chemical procedure [6] and shown that a mean of 83% (standard deviation 6.8%) of the total protein in 13 successive preparations was interferon protein.

A key point in the large-scale production of interferon from Namalwa cells is to ensure uniformly high titers in the crude product. This can be achieved by routinely treating the cells with sodium butyrate before inducing formation of interferon [7].

In a dose-tolerance study in man [8], the side-effects with our lymphoblastoid cell interferon were essentially the same as after administration of Finnish leukocyte interferon. There was a dose-dependent febrile response to the first one or two i.m. injections and a longer course resulted in leukopenia, lassitude, and malaise. When injected intravenously into rabbits, the interferon preparations also led to rises in their body temperatures, but with a time course unlike that seen with bacterial endotoxin. The pyrogenicity in rabbits and man of different preparations was proportional to the amount of interferon injected, and did not correlate with the very low contents of endotoxin measured by the Limulus amoebocyte lysate test. The febrile response in man was comparable to that observed after injections of an equivalent number of units of considerably less pure preparations of buffy-coat cell interferon. We conclude that leukocyte interferons are intrinsically pyrogenic in man and rabbits.

Workers in several laboratories now have clones of bacteria expressing interferon genes, and we ourselves have access to such clones. Nevertheless, although we are at present probably the largest producer of interferon for clinical use, we are currently increasing our capability for making lymphoblastoid interferon. We feel strongly that this is worthwhile for the following reasons.

First, all the chemical, physical, biological, and human dose-tolerance data suggest that the purified interferons we obtain from Namalwa cells resemble those made by buffy-coat cells. It is therefore likely that in clinical use, the results with our interferon will mirror those already seen with buffy-coat cell interferon.

Second, chemical analysis has shown that our preparations contain at least 8 different interferon proteins, the product of at least 5 structural genes, and at least some of these differ in their antigenic and biological properties from others [*D. C. Burke,* personal communication]. Each bacterial clone with an inserted human interferon gene will make only one interferon; such individual interferon proteins also differ from one another and from the natural mixture of leukocyte interferons derived from human white-blood cells in their biological effects [9]. It will take considerable time to determine whether any one such interferon protein, or even mixtures of two or three, will mimic in man the full range of antitumor and antiviral activity provided by the natural mixture. In such studies it will be important to have a human white-cell product as a benchmark, and we believe our lymphoblastoid-cell preparations can provide this. It should be noted that some antitumor activity was seen in our Phase-I study [8], and recent results, to be presented in detail elsewhere, have shown antitumor activity in further patients with malignant melanoma. Studies in other forms of cancer are in progress, but it is too early for the results to be assessed.

Third, the limited availability, thus far, of interferons made from human cells has led many to suppose that recombinant DNA technology offers the only possible way of making adequate amounts of interferon available at a reasonable cost. We do not support this view. Our production costs have fallen significantly as the scale of our production has increased, and can be expected to decrease further (our production tanks are very large in terms of current tissue-culture technology, but still small compared with those routinely used in antibiotic fermentation). It is likely that the cost of the crude interferon, whether made from cultured cells or from bacteria, will ultimately form a very small proportion of the total cost of the final bottled, tested, and distributed product. Thus it is on its clinical performance that the choice of an interferon preparation should be made. If Namalwa-cell interferon proves to have clinical advantages, it can certainly be prepared in quantities adequate for very wide-spread use.

References

1 Strander, H.; Cantell, K.: Production of Interferon by Human Leukocytes in Vitro. Ann/s Med. exp. Biol. Fenn. *44:*265 (1966).

2 Strander, H.; Mogensen, K. E.; Cantell, K.: production of human lymphoblastoid interferon. J. clin. Microbiol. *1:*116 – 124 (1975).

3 Christofinis, G. J.; Steel, C. M.; Finter, N. B.: Interferon production by human lymphoblastoid cell lines of different origins. J. gen. Virol. *52:*169 – 171, (1981).

4 Finter, N. B.; Fantes, K. H.: The purity and safety of interferons prepared for clinical use: The case for lymphoblastoid interferon. Interferon *2:*65 – 79 (1980).

5 Allen, G.; Fantes, K. H.: A family of structural genes for human lymphoblastoid (leukocyte-type) interferon. Nature *287:*408 – 411 (1980).

6 Fantes, K. H.; Allen, G.: The specific activity of pure human interferons and a non-biological method for estimating the purity of highly purified interferon preparations. J. Interferon Res. (in press, 1981).

7 Johnston, M. D.: Improvement in or relating to a process for producing interferon. European Patent Application 78100395.9 (1979).

8 Priestman, T. J.: Initial evaluation of human lymphoblastoid interferon in patients with advanced malignant disease. Lancet *ii*: 113 – 118 (1980).

9 Yelverton, E.: Leung, D.; Weck, P.; Gray, P. W.; Goeddel, D. V.: Bacterial synthesis of novel human leukocyte interferon. Nucl. Acids Res. *9:*731 – 741 (1981).

Dr. N. B. Finter, Virology Research & Development Department, Wellcome Research Laboratories, Langley Court, Beckenham, GB-Kent

Production of Human Gamma Interferon for Clinical Trials[1]

Peter von Wussow, Michelle Chen, Chris D. Platsoucas, Marzenna Wiranowska-Stewart, William E. Stewart II

Memorial Sloan-Kettering Cancer Center, New York, N. Y., USA

Introduction

Several studies have suggested that gamma interferons have activity potentials distinct from those exerted by the alpha and beta interferons. Initially, *Salvin et al.* [10] demonstrated that crude preparations of murine IFN-γ were able to induce antitumor activities in mice at dose levels several 100-fold below doses of murine IFN-α/β required to detect antitumor effects. This report was supported by other studies of similar dose-discrepancies for antitumor activities of α/β vs IFN-γ preparations [2]. Further, IFN-γ preparations have been reported to exert markedly potent anticellular activities in vitro [1, 9], in some cases acting on cells that are completely resistant to any of the activities of α and β to IFNs [8]. Also our work has suggested that HuIFN-γ has different receptors than HuIFN-α and β [12], and some studies suggest that IFN-γ may synergize the activity of IFNs α and β ([7] and Y. K. Yip, personal communication, 1981).

Such studies make it tempting to specualte that IFN-γ may be a more potent antitumor/immunomodulatory agent than IFNs-α/β. However, to date no one has provided any convincing data that it is the IFN-γ in these preparations that is responsible for these activities and, obviously, such relatively crude preparations contain numerous other lymphokines able to exert a variety of activities. Attempts at

[1] Supported in part by Grant No. AI-16439 from the USPHS-NIAID. William E. Stewart II was supported by Research Career Development Award AI-00219 from the NIH-NIAID. Peter von Wussow was supported by Deutsche Forschungsgemeinschaft.

achieving highly purified preparations of IFN-γ have been frustrated, as always, by the lack of adequate starting materials and by the remarkable instability of these materials purified to any significant extent.

On the one hand, it is important to ascertain whether the IFN-γ is the active component in such preparations. On the other hand, it is also important to determine whether even crude preparations are clinically interesting, even if the IFN in them is not the responsible agent. Therefore, we have undertaken to make HuIFN-γ preparations sufficiently purified so that they contain no toxic inducer, yet stable enough for reliable dose estimations. We have found that this cannot be achieved using staphylococcal enterotoxins but can be accomplished by inducing lymphocytes with specific antibodies.

Materials and Methods

Mitogens

Phytohemagglutinin purified (PHA-P; Wellcome Research Laboratories, Beckenham, U. K.), concanavalin A (Sigma Chemicals, St. Louis Missouri) or pokeweed mitogen (Sigma Chemicals) were used at optimal inducing doses of 3 μg, 5 μg, and 10 μg, respectively. Staphylococcal enterotoxin A (SEA) was provided by the U.S.F.D.A. (Cincinatti, Ohio) and was used at 0.02 μg/ml. Staphylococcal enterotoxin B (SEB), from Sigma Chemicals, was used at 0.02 μg.

Monoclonal Antibodies and Heterologous Antisera

OKT_3, OKT_4, and OKT_8 monoclonal antibodies were obtained from Ortho Pharmaceutical Corp. (Raritan, N. J.). OKT_3 were used at several concentrations as described in the text; OKT_4 and OKT_8 were employed at 600 μg/ml and 1200 μg/ml. Anti-human Lyt1, anti-human Lyt2, anti-human Lyt3, and anti-human Ia monoclonal antibody (New England Nuclear, Boston, Massachusetts) were used at concentrations of 0.25, 2.5, 12.5, and 25 μg per ml. Anti-T-cell antibody, purchased from Hybritech (La Jolla, California), was evaluated at dilution ratios from 1 : 10 to 1 : 10000. Anti-HLA monoclonal antibody (clone W6/32 HLK) as well as anti-β_2-microglobulin monoclonal antibody (clone 26/114 HLK), from Accurate Chemicals and Scientific Corp. (Hillsville, New York) were tested at concentrations of 0.002, 2, and 0.2 mg/ml and 0.5, 5, and 50 μg/ml, respectively. Rabbit anti-Ia-serum was kindly provided by Dr. S. Cunningham-Rundles of this Center and was used at final dilution ratios of 1 : 10, 1 : 100, and 1 : 1000. Anti-lymphocyte serum from Hyland (Glendale, California) was employed at final dilution ratios of 1 : 10, 1 : 20, 1 : 60, and 1 : 80. Anti-Ig + IgA + IgM + IgD from Miles (Yeda, Israel) was evaluated at dilution ratios of 1 : 10, 1 : 100, 1 : 1000. Anti-thymocyte-globulin, provided by Upjohn Corp., was tested at final dilution ratios of 1 : 10, 1 : 100, 1 : 1000, 1 : 10000.

Preparations of Cells

Fresh human peripheral leukocytes obtained from healthy human subjects were mixed with phosphate-buffered saline (PBS) and 6% hydroxy-methyl starch (Volex Hepastarch) at a ratio of 2 : 1 : 1. After 2 h at room temperature the cells of the upper layer were harvested, washed twice, and resuspended in RPMI-1640 medium containing 1% glutamine and 2% fetal bovine serum (FBS) at a concentration of 5×10^6 cells/ml.

Interferon Inductions and Assays

Peripheral blood leukocyte suspensions (5×10^6 cells/ml) were cultured in RPMI-1640 medium containing 1% glutamine and 2% FBS. The cells were incubated with the various inducers either in 5 ml plastic tubes or in 96-well microtiter plates (Falcon) for 3 days at 37°C in a humidified 5% CO_2 atmosphere. Cell-free supernatant fluids were tested for IFN activity.

IFN titrations were done by a microassay based on inhibition of the pathogenic effect of VSV [11]. All samples were tested on human fibroblasts trisomic for chromosome 21, on human WISH cells, and on bovine kidney cells (MDBK). On every 96-well plate a laboratory standard human alpha-IFN calibrated against the National Institutes of Health standard for IFN- (G-023-901-527, N.I.H.) was assayed. The IFN-γ levels of test supernatants were not adjusted to the IFN-α reference.

Anti-Interferon Antisera

Anti-serum to HuIFN-α titrating about 60000 HuIFN-α neutralizing units/ml, was kindly provided by Dr. Kari Cantell (Central Public Health Laboratory, Helsinki, Finland). Antiserum to HuIFN-β was a generous gift of Dr. Jan Vilcek (New York University, New York, N.Y.), and titrated 15000 HuIFN-β neutralization units/ml.

Purification Methods

Interferon preparations induced by SEA and by antibodies were routinely purified by chromatography on controlled pore glass (CPG 350-B mesh size 120/200, Electronucleonics Inc., Fairfield, N. J.) as previously described [13]. HuIFN-γ eluted in 0.02 M phosphate buffer, pH 7.2 + 20% ethylene glycol in 1 M NaCl.

HuIFN-γ eluted from CPG was dialyzed against 30 mM NH_4HCO_3 (pH 7.6), lyophilized, resuspended in PBS, applied to a column of Sephadex G-100, and eluted with the same buffer. Interferon-gamma activity-peak eluted from the Sephadex G-100 column was applied directly to a column of concanavalin A-Sepharose (Pharmacia) and was eluted with 25 mM α-methyl-mannoside (α-MM), 50 mM "α-MM, 100 mM α-MM, and 1M NaCl + 50% ethylene glycol.

Results

Monoclonal anti-human T-cell antibody OKT_3, which recognizes the majority (85%) of the peripheral blood E-rosetting cells, induced IFN-γ production in suspensions of human leukocytes (table I); however, OKT_4 antibody, which recognizes an antigen expressed on a subpopulation (65%) of T-cells containing helper activity, induced

Table I. Induction of human gamma interferon by antibodies and mitogens

Inducer	IFN titer (units/ml)
Anti-lymphocyte serum	1000–2000
Anti-thymocyte serum	1000–2000
OKT_3 antibodies	100–1000
OKT_4 antibodies	10–60
OKT_8 antibodies	<10
Anti-HuLyt 3	<10
Anti-HuLyt 2	<10
Anti-HuLyt 1	<10
Anti-T-cell (Hybritech)	<10
Anti-HLA (Sera Lab)	<10
Anti-β_2-microglobulin (Sera Lab)	<10
Anti-Ia serum	<10
Anti-IgG A-M-D serum	<10
SEA	1000
PWM	1000
Con-A	300
PHA	300

only marginal IFN-γ production. OKT_8 monoclonal antibody, which defines a subpopulation of cells containing lymphocytes with cytotoxic/suppressor functions, failed to induce IFN-γ. Both a horse anti-human thymocyte globulin and a goat anti-human lymphocytic serum were good interferon inducers. Several other monoclonal antibodies (e.g. HuLyt-3, HuLyt-2, HuLyt-1, and anti-T-cell antibodies) recognizing the SRBC receptor(s) or antigens expressed on some of the E-rosetting cells were also evaluated for induction of IFN-γ, but none of these were able to induce IFN-γ at any of the concentrations tested. Furthermore, monoclonal anti-HLA and anti-β_2-microglobulin antibodies as well as heterologous anti-Ig and anti-Ia antibodies failed to induce IFN-γ.

The IFN levels induced by the different inducers varied from donor to donor, but similar amounts of antiviral activity were induced by either staphylococcus enterotoxin A, pokeweed mitogen, or the antisera ALS and ATS. OKT_3, PHA, and Con-A elicited only slightly lower levels of IFN in these cultures.

Supernatant fluids from various cell cultures induced by either SEA, SEB, OKT_3, ALS, or ATS were assayed on various human fibroblasts and on bovine kidney cells; only the human fibroblasts

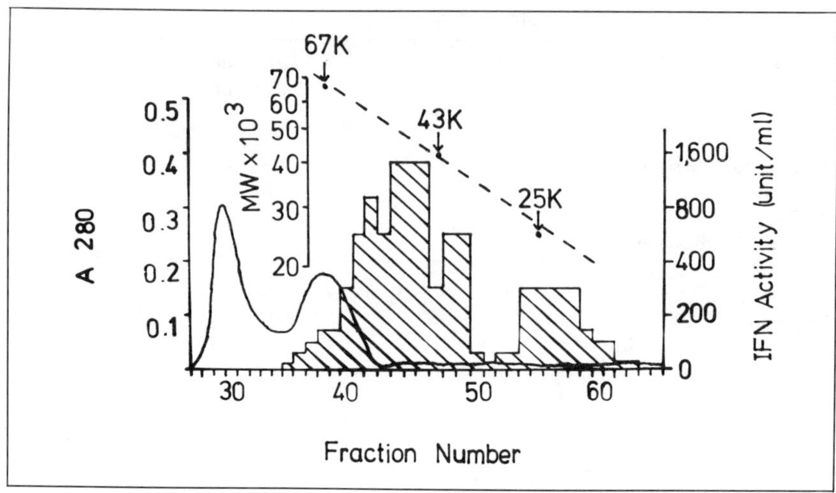

Figure 1. Purification of human gamma interferon by Sephadex G-100 chromatography. HuIFN-γ preparation containing about $10^{5.0}$ units previously purified to approximately $10^{4.3}$ units/mg protein by chromatography on controlled pore glass was applied to Sephadex G-100 in PBS and eluted in this buffer. Recovery was approximately 80% at approximately $10^{5.5}$ units/mg protein.

were protected against vesicular stomatitis virus. The antiviral activity was not neutralized by antisera recognizing either human IFN-α or IFN-β. The interferon was unstable to overnight treatment at pH 2. Therefore, this interferon fulfills the criteria of human IFN-γ.

Interferon induced by SEA or antibodies can be purified by CPG chromatography to a specific activity of about 10^4 units/mg protein with virtually 100% recovery of activity ([13] and unpublished data). This interferon can be further purified by sizing-filtration through Sephadex G-100 (fig. 1), again with satisfactory recovery of activity, ranging from 30 to 70% and a specific activity of about $10^{5.5}$ to $10^{6.0}$ units/mg protein. This material can be dialyzed against NH_4HCO_3 buffer and lyophilized and is stable in this form to prolonged storage [*M. Chen et al.*, unpublished data]. Such sizing separation is sufficient to eliminate the antibody-inducer molecules from the HuIFN-γ (approximately 45000 daltons) but the SEA (about 30000 daltons) is inefficiently resolved by this method. In fact, we have found that the material induced by SEA still contains significant levels of the in-

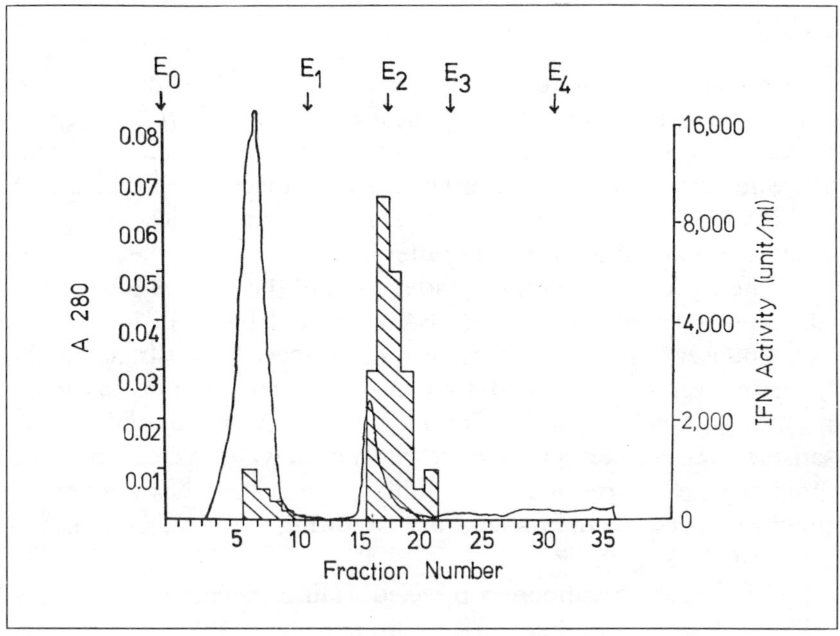

Figure 2. Purification of human gamma interferon by concanavalin A-Sepharose chromatography. HuIFN-γ preparation containing about 10^5 units previously purified to approximately $10^{5.5}$ units/mg protein by sequential chromatography on CPG and Sephadex G-100 was applied to the concanavalin A-Sepharose in PBS (E_0) and eluted with 25 mM α-MM (E_1), 50 mM α-MM (E_2), 100 mM α-MM (E_3), and 1 M naCl + 50% ethylene glycol (E_4). Recovery was approximately 70% at > 10^6/mg protein.

ducer after purification on CPG and Sephadex, which could be detected by the ability of SEA to elevate human natural-killer cell activity [*C. Platsoucas et al.*, unpublished data].

Therefore, it was deemed necessary to purify such SEA-induced HuIFN-γ preparations further to attempt to eliminate this residual inducer. This could be accomplished by chromatography on concanavalin A-Sepharose (fig. 2), which yielded material purified much in excess of 10^6 units/mg of protein. However, accurate calculations of either percentage recovery or specific activities are difficult from such column runs, apparently due to the marked lability of highly purified material, which resulted in losses of several orders of magnitude either on storage or further processing.

Discussion

Human gamma interferon can be induced in peripheral blood leukocytes by a number of mitogenic agents. The *Falcoffs* first reported induction of human IFN-γ by antilymphocytic serum more than 10 years ago [3 – 6]. Subsequently, several mitogenic substances such as PHA were also found to induce HuIFN-γ. Apparently, it was the relative easier availability of the latter inducers that diverted attention from the use of the "immune" inducers, and the relative low cost of the staphylococcal enterotoxin, SEA, seems to have made it attractive as an inducer of HuIFN-γ. However, our studies demonstrate that the latter inducer is difficult to eliminate from preparations, as it copurifies on CPG and its resolution in sizing chromatography is not satisfactory. Further purification on concanavalin-A may help remove some of the residual toxin inducer, but such extensive purification introduces severe problems of loss, owing to the marked instability of the HuIFN-γ.

Using specific antibodies directed against T-lymphocytes (ALS, ATS, monoclonal antibody OKT_3) we have been able to induce approximately the same levels of HuIFN-γ as induced by the staphylococcal enterotoxins. These preparations could be purified by CPG chromatography and sizing separation, to eliminate the inducer, at a specific activity where the final product will be stable to processing and storage. Such HuIFN-γ preparations should be acceptable for clinical trials to determine whether such gamma interferon-containing preparations indeed have potent immunomodulatory and antitumor activities in man.

References

1 Blalock, J. E.; Georgiades, J. A.; Langford, M. P.; Johnson, H. M.: Purified human immune interferon has more potent anticellular activity than fibroblast or leukocyte interferon. Cell. Immunol. *49:*390 – 394 (1980).

2 Crane, J. L.; Glasgow, L. A.; Kern, E. R.; Youngner, J. S.: Inhibition of murine osteogenic sarcoma by treatment with type I or type II interferon. J. natn. Cancer Inst. *61:*871 – 874 (1978).

3 Falcoff, E.; Falcoff, R.; Eyquem, A.; Sanceau, J.; Catinot, L.; Vomecourt, A.: Induction d'interferon humain par le serum antilymphocytaire. C. r. Acad. Sci. *271 D:*545 – 549 (1970).

4 Falcoff, E.; Falcoff, R.; Catinot, L.; Vomecourt, A.; Sanceau, J.: Synthesis of interferon in human lymphocytes stimulated in vitro by antilymphocytic serum. Revue eur. Etud. clin. biol. *17:*20 – 26 (1972).

5 Falcoff, R.: Some properties of virus and immune-induced human lymphocyte interferons. J. gen. Virol. *16:* 251 – 253 (1972).

6 Falcoff, R.; Oriol, R.; Iscaki, S.: Lymphocyte stimulation and interferon induction by 7S anti-human leukocyte globulins and their uni- and divalent fragments. Eur. J. Immunol. *2:* 476 – 478 (1972).

7 Fleischmann, W. R.; Georgiades, J. A.; Osborne, L. C.; Johnson, H. M.: Potentiation of interferon activity by mixed preparations of fibroblast and immune interferon. Infect. Immunity *26:* 248 – 253 (1979).

8 Hovanessian, A. G.; La Bonnardiere, C.; Falcoff, E.: Action of murine-γ (immune) interferon on β (fibroblast) interferon-resistant L1210 and embryonal carcinoma cells. J. Interferon Res. *1:* 125 – 136 (1980).

9 Rubin, B. Y.; Gupta, S. L.: Differential efficacies of human type I and type II interferons as antiviral and antiproliferative agents. Proc. natn. Acad. Sci. USA *77:* 5928 – 5932 (1980).

10 Salvin, S. B.; Youngner, J. S.; Nishio, J.; Neta, R.: Tumor suppression by a lymphokine released into the circulation of mice with delayed hypersensitivity. J. natn. Cancer Inst. *55:* 1233 – 1237 (1975).

11 Stewart, W. E., II: The Interferon System (Springer-Verlag, Vienna 1979).

12 Stewart, W. E., II; Wiranowska-Stewart, M.: Relative sensitivities of human cells to interferon types I and II: The role of chromosome 21. Abstr. annu. Meet. Am. Soc. Microbiol. (Abstract) T8 (1980).

13 Wiranowska-Stewart, M.; Lin, L. S.; Braude, I. A.; Stewart, W. E., II: Production, partial purification, and characterization of human and murine interferons – type II. Molec. Immunol. *17:* 625 – 633 (1980).

Prof. Dr. W. E. Stewart, II, Interferon Laboratory, Memorial Sloan-Kettering Cancer Center, 1275 York Avenue, USA-New York 10021, N.Y.

Immune Interferon Production by T-Cell Clones

Peter H. Krammer[1]; *Ursula Kees*[1]; *Fabrizio Marcucci*[2], *Holger Kirchner*[2]

[1] Institut für Immunologie und Genetik, Deutsches Krebsforschungszentrum, Heidelberg, FRG

[2] Institut für Virusforschung, Deutsches Krebsforschungszentrum, Heidelberg, FRG

Introduction

Interferon (IFN) has been discovered more than 20 years ago by *Isaacs* and *Lindenmann* through its inhibitory effect on viral replication. Since then it became obvious that a number of pleiotropic effects could be attributed to different IFN proteins [4]. Thus, in man several leukocyte IFN (IFN-α) could be distinguished from fibroblast-(IFN-β) and immune IFN (IFN-γ). IFN-α can be produced by leukocytes by a variety of stimuli (e.g. virus); IFN-β is released from fibroblasts, and IFN-γ is produced by lymphocytes during the course of an immune response [10, 3]. For many years it has been difficult to study the biological effects of IFN as preparations of purified IFN in sufficient quantity were not available. The reason for this was because IFN was produced from most cells but only in low quantities. Over the last few years, however, at least with respect to IFN-α and IFN-β, the situation has changed considerably. Cell lines were found which could be stimulated towards "superproduction", and with gene technology the IFN-α and -β genes could be introduced into E. coli bacteria which then produced large quantities of IFN-α and -β. This lead to the determination of the protein sequence of IFN-α and -β as well as the nucleotide sequence of the coding genes [2, 6, 8, 9]. Products from such cell lines or bacteria are now increasingly used to study the biology of IFN.

The above only applies to IFN-α and -β. Although IFN-γ had been discovered as a lymphokine in 1965 [10], comparatively little progress has been made with respect to the definition of the IFN-γ producer cell or IFN-γ purification. This is most probably due to the fact that the immune system is a complex mixture of interacting cells which, under the available conditions, produce IFN-γ only in relatively small quantities. The experiments described in this paper define the IFN-γ producer cells and describe the methods by which high quantities of IFN-γ can be obtained from such cells.

Analysis of IFN-γ Production from T-Cells in Limiting Dilution Microcultures

To determine the IFN-γ producer cells, their frequency and range of activities, we designed the following experimental system. Murine spleen cells, stimulated by the T-cell mitogen Concanavalin-A (Con-A), were, for 2 days, Ficoll purified, plated in limiting dilution, and further expanded for 7 to 12 days in the presence of irradiated peritoneal exudate filler cells and medium substituted with T-cell growth factors (TCGF). With a low cell number of 1, 2, 4, etc. cells per well initially plated clone sizes of several 100 to several 1000 cells could be reached. On a statistical basis a high percentage of cultures could be obtained with cells derived from one or few precursor cells. The clone sizes were sufficient for the cells to be tested in functional assays. The cells from each microculture were thoroughly washed to remove any contaminating TCGF and stimulated by Con-A for 24 h to produce IFN-γ and other lymphokines into the supernatant. In addition, samples of cells from each microculture well could be simultaneously and directly tested, e.g. for total non-specific cytolytic activity on EL4 tumor target cells in the presence of Con-A to attach the killer to the target cells. This system provided a new method to assess the whole spectrum of T-cell activities and lymphokines released from T-cells responsive to the mitogen Con-A. Our experiments gave the following results:

(1) IFN-γ release and the production of other lymphokines was not constitutive but could only be obtained upon induction;
(2) IFN-γ was produced by cytotoxic and noncytotoxic T-cells;
(3) cultures with the most potent cytolytic activity gave the highest IFN-γ titers; and
(4) individual selected microcultures containing 10^4 to 5×10^4 cells yielded titers of IFN-γ above 10^4 IU [5].

Since the frequency estimates for cells producing other lymphokine-like colony-stimulating factors (CSF) [*Staber et al.,* to be published] were even higher than those for IFN-γ, these data suggested that most T-cells produce IFN-γ, and that the IFN-γ-producing fraction of T-cells overlapped with the fraction of T-cells producing CSF, i.e., one T-cell could release several lymphokines at the same time. Furthermore, under culture conditions bypassing regulation and growth control normally operative in cell mixtures of bulk cultures, very high titers could be obtained. This implies a stringent regulatory system for IFN-γ and the production of other T-cell lymphokines. For practical purposes it allows us to define an IFN-γ producer cell which provides a high yield for further biochemical analysis.

Analysis of IFN-γ Production from T-Cell Clones in Long-Term Culture

Almost invariably T-cell clones from primary cultures (see above) die in medium substituted with TCGF alone and cannot be propagated in long-term cultures over a period of three weeks. A low incidence of long-term T-cell cultures growing in medium and TCGF was observed [1]. We derived such long-term lines from cultures of antigen-activated T-cells and cloned these lines by limiting dilution. A large number of clones with stable growth properties and a doubling time of approximately 20 h were obtained. These clones could easily be frozen and thawed and several of them have by now been maintained in permanent culture for more than 1½ years. Preliminary data on the cell surface markers of some clones indicated that T-cell markers were only expressed on some clones while other clones appeared as null cells or may have lost such markers. We decided to use these clones to test similar parameters as with T-cells plated in short-term limiting dilution microcultures. Similar data as described above were obtatined. T-cell clones from long-term cultures produced IFN-γ in the absence of adherent cells upon induction with T- and not B-cell mitogens. Some of these clones yielded high quantities of IFN-γ which have never been obtained from cell mixtures in bulk cultures [7]. Several subclones of an IFN-γ high-producer clone isolated by single-cell manipulation produced IFN-γ, CSF, and MAF (macrophage activating factor) at the same time [*Kees et al.,* to be published].

This provides evidence that at least certain T-cells are capable of simultaneously producing several lymphokines upon an inductive stimulus.

Regulation of IFN-γ and Lymphokine Activity

We conclude that T-cells produce IFN-γ in variable quantities upon an inductive T-cell-specific signal and that it can also produce different lymphokines like IFN-γ, CSF and MAF simultaneously. We may assume that a particular T-cell can produce an even larger number of lymphokines. Since some of these lymphokines exert their apparent activities on different target cells, the following questions arise:

(1) Are some of the lymphokines, as defined by different assay systems, actually different molecules?
(2) Could a given lymphokine have different activities at different molecular concentrations?
(3) Do some of the lymphokines belong to a family of structurally related molecules which have evolved from a common precursor?
(4) Are the genes, coding for some of the lymphokines, arranged in tandem so that a common inductive signal is sufficient to trigger the transcription of several of them simultaneously?
(5) What is the physiological signal to induce lymphokine release?
(6) What is the biological function of the lymphokines, and is it different from the activity in the assay systems which define them?
(7) What are the possible mechanisms of regulating lymphokine activity?

This list of questions is by far not complete and shall only serve to stimulate further experiments to elucidate the role of lymphokines including IFN-γ. This short discussion will be limited and address several possible aspects of the last question only.

Different lymphokines, when produced upon an inductive signal during an immune response from the same T-cell, are potent effector molecules. They are active in minute quantities on a variety of target cells in different anatomical locations. This implies a stringent regulatory control on their activity. In principle, several possibilities for regulation could exist:

(a) regulation of the lymphokine production at the level of the producer cells, i.e. by alterating the rate of production or by stimulating or inhibiting clonal expansion of the producer cells;

(b) regulation by direct activation or inactivation of the lymphokines; and

(c) regulation of activity on the target-cell level, e.g. by competitive mechanisms.

It is conceivable that these possibilities are not merely alternatives but might coexist. Since the immune system has developed mechanisms of regulation, effectively exerted by different T-cell compartments, one could postulate that, within this frame, lymphokines and their antagonists might also be released from different T-cells.

It is obvious that new experimental protocols might be needed to gain further insight into these complex regulatory processes. It is not unreasonable to predict that IFN-γ, as a lymphokine with a reproducible and quantifiable activity, might serve as a useful guide to the "lymphokine world".

References

1 V. Boehmer, H.; Haas, W.: H-2-restricted cytolytic and noncytolytic T-cell clones: Isolation, specificity, and functional analysis. Immunol. Rev. *54:* 27–56 (1981).

2 Derynck, R.; Content, J.; DeClercq, E.; Volckaert, G.; Tavernier, J.; Devos, R.; Fiers, W.: Isolation and structure of a human fibroblast interferon gene. Nature *285:* 542–546 (1980).

3 Gifford, G. E.; Tibor, A.; Peavy, D. L.: Interferon production in mixed lymphocyte cell cultures. Infect. Immunity *3:* 164–166 (1971).

4 Gresser, I.; De Mayer-Guignard, J.; Tovey, M. G.; De Mayer, E.: Electrophoretically pure mouse interferon exerts multiple biologic effects. Proc. natn. Acad. Sci. *76:* 5308–5312 (1979).

5 Krammer, P. H.; Marcucci, F.; Waller, M.; Kirchner, H.: Heterogeneity of soluble T-cell products. I. Frequency and correlation analysis of cytotoxic and immune interferon (IFN-γ) producing spleen cells in the mouse (manuscript submitted).

6 Mantei, N.; Schwarzstein, M.; Streuli, M.; Panem, S.; Nagata, S.; Weissmann, C.: The nucleotide sequence of a clonal human leukocyte interferon DNA. Gene *10:* 1–10 (1980).

7 Marcucci, F.; Waller, M.; Kirchner, H.; Krammer, P. H.: Production of immune interferon by murine T-cell clones from long-term cultures. Nature *291:* 79–81 (1981).

8 Taniguchi, T.; Mantei, N.; Schwarzstein, M.; Nagata, S.; Muramatsu, M.; Weissmann, C.: Human leukocyte and fibroblast interferons are structurally related. Nature *285:* 547–549 (1980).

9 Taniguchi, T.; Ohno, S.; Fujii-Kuriyama, Y.; Maramatsu, M.: The nucleotide sequence of human fibroblast interferon cDNA. Gene *10:* 11 – 15 (1980).
10 Wheelock, E. F.: Interferon-like virus inhibitor in human leukocytes by phytohemagglutinin. Science *149:*310 – 311 (1965).

Dr. Peter Krammer, PD, Institut für Immunologie und Genetik, Deutsches Krebsforschungszentrum, Im Neuenheimer Feld 280, D-6900 Heidelberg

Induction and Characterization of Human Immune (Gamma) Interferon

J. Vilček, Y. K. Yip, R. H. L. Pang[1]

Department of Microbiology, New York University School of Medicine, New York, N.Y., USA

Introduction

Immune interferon, termed IFN-γ according to the recently adopted official terminology [1], still remains the least well-characterized IFN species. For a number of reasons a great deal of interest is being focused on IFN-γ. At least one of the reasons for this interest undoubtedly has to do with the simple fact that so little is known about its properties and activities. Exploring and conquering new frontiers has always provided one of the major excitements in scientific life.

There are, however, some other good reasons for the very keen interest in IFN-γ. Thus, preliminary evidence suggests that IFN-γ may be more active than IFN-α and IFN-β in its immunoregulatory and cell growth inhibitory activities [2–4]. It appears that the molecular mechanisms of action of IFN-γ are somewhat different from the other IFNs [3, 5, 6]. It has also been shown that simultaneous treatment of some cells with IFN-γ and IFN-α or IFN-β may result in a mutually potentiating cooperative effect [7]. These findings form the basis for the belief that the clinical efficacy of IFN-γ in patients with malignancies may be superior to that of the other available IFNs.

One of the major problems in working with IFN-γ has been the lack of efficient and reproducible methods for its production. Without a good supply of suitable starting material, purification was an

[1] Present address: Genex Corporation, Rockville, MD 20852, USA

insurmountable task. Development of efficient induction methods is also a prerequisite for the successful isolation of IFN-γ mRNA and the cloning of IFN-γ complementary DNA.

Several methods of IFN-γ production have been described since the original demonstration by *Wheelock* [8] that production of a new IFN species could be induced in human lymphocytes by stimulation with phytohemagglutinin (PHA). All published methods of IFN-γ production are based on the stimulation of cultured lymphocytes with mitogens, including various lectins [8, 9], staphylococcal enterotoxin-A [10], antilymphocyte serum [11] or other stimuli [12–14]. However, the yields of IFN-γ produced with these mitogens are quite variable and often rather low.

Enhancement of Human IFN-γ Production by TPA and Related Compounds

Recently we developed a quite reproducible method of human IFN-γ production based on the combined stimulation of lymphocyte cultures with a lectin (usually PHA) and the phorbol ester, 12-0-tetradecanoylphorbol-13-acetate (TPA). TPA itself is known to be a T-cell mitogen and, in addition, it is capable of enhancing the mitogenic activity of several lectins in lymphocytes [15, 16]. In earlier studies, TPA was also shown to enhance spontaneous IFN-α production in lymphocytes [17]. These findings prompted us to examine the effect of TPA on PHA-induced IFN-γ production in human lymphocyte cultures [18, 19].

Treatment of lymphocytes with TPA alone can result in the production of low levels of IFN. Treatment with PHA alone in many instances also results in the production of rather low levels of IFN. Combined stimulation with TPA and PHA quite reproducibly leads to the production of IFN yields that are far in excess of the sum of the yields obtained by separate stimulation with the two agents alone (table I).

Similar results were obtained by combined stimulation with TPA and many other mitogens, including various lectins (e.g., concanavalin-A, wheat-germ agglutinin, pokeweed mitogen), staphylococcal enterotoxin-A, staphylococcal protein-A, galactose oxidase, and other agents previously shown to act as inducers of IFN-γ. IFN production

Table I. Interferon production in human leukocyte cultures after combined stimulation with TPA and PHA[1]

TPA	IFN units/ml at PHA concentration (μg/ml)			
ng/ml	0	5	10	25
0	<40	120	80	160
5	40	2,560	1,280	960
25	480	3,840	1,920	1,280
50	160	2,560	2,560	1,280
75	240	5,120	1,920	1,280
100	120	3,840	3,840	1,920

[1] Cultures were seeded with unseparated cells from lymphocyte-rich plateletpheresis residues at a concentration of 2×10^6 leukocytes/ml in serum-free RPMI 1640 medium. TPA was added to cultures at the time of seeding; 2 h later PHA was added at the indicated concentrations. IFN yields were determined in culture fluids collected after 48 h incubation at 37°C.

was demonstrated after stimulation of human lymphocyte cultures with any of these agents alone, and this production was significantly enhanced by co-stimulation of cultures with TPA. These results are reported in detail elsewhere [20].

A number of TPA analogues have also been examined for their ability to enhance IFN production in cultures of human peripheral lymphocytes. TPA is a potent tumor-promoting agent when tested in the 2-stage mouse skin carcinogenesis assay [21]. It was of interest to determine whether there was a correlation between tumor-promoting and IFN production-enhancing activities of various TPA analogues and related compounds. As shown in table II, the correlation between these activities is not perfect. In addition to TPA, two other diterpene esters were found to act as potent enhancers of IFN production at the low concentration of 5ng/ml. One of these, the plant-derived ester mezerein, was at least as potent as TPA in stimulating IFN production while known to be essentially devoid of tumor-promoting activity. In contrast, phorbol-12,13-didecanoate was less potent as an enhancer of IFN production, while known to be highly active as a tumor-promoting agent. A structurally unrelated tumor-promoting agent, teleocidin [22] was also found to have IFN-stimulating activity (not shown).

The finding that mezerein, although lacking significant tumor-promoting activity, is at least as potent as TPA in stimulating IFN

Table II. Comparison of IFN-stimulating, tumor-promoting, and inflammatory activities of various diterpene esters

Compound	IFN-stimulating activity at ng/ml[1]		Activity on mouse skin[2]	
	5	500	Tumor-promoting	Inflammatory
Phorbol	–	–	–	–
4α-phorbol	–	–	–	–
4α-phorbol 12,13-didecanoate	–	–	–	–
Phorbol 13,20-diacetate	–	–	–	–
Phorbol 12-monomyristate	–	+	–	–
Phorbol 12,13-diacetate	–	+	+	+
Phorbol 12,13-dibenzoate	–	+	+	+
Phorbol 12,13-didecanoate	–	+	+	+
Phorbol 12,13-dibutyrate	+	+	+	+
Phorbol 12-myristate-13-acetate (TPA)	+	+	+	+
Mezerein	+	+	–	+

[1] As determined by enhancement of PHA-stimulated IFN production in cultures of human peripheral white blood cells [20].
[2] Based on published data [21] and information provided by the manufacturer.
Symbols: +, positive; ±, weakly positive; –, negative.

production [20], could be exploited for the production of IFN for clinical application. This approach is now being actively pursued by some laboratories in the U.S.A. IFN produced in lymphocyte cultures by combined stimulation with TPA or mezerein and PHA shows properties characteristic for IFN-γ (see below).

Induction of IFN-γ by Monoclonal Antibody OKT3, Reactive with Human Lymphocytes

Several years ago *Falcoff et al.* [11] showed that antilymphocyte serum in the absence of complement acted as an inducer of IFN-γ in cultures of human mononuclear cells. More recently, *Van Wauwe et al.* [23] demonstrated that monoclonal antibody OKT3, reactive with a surface component of all mature human T-cells [24], exerted a potent mitogenic effect in T-lymphocytes. These findings prompted us to examine the IFN-inducing capacity of OKT3 antibody (table III).

Table III. IFN induction with monoclonal antibody OKT3 in cultures of plateletpheresis residues from different donors[1]

OKT3-antibody concentration (ng/ml)	IFN units/ml from unit No.			
	I	II	III	IV
1	< 40	<40	40	5,120
2	< 40	<40	240	10,240
5	160	60	1,280	15,360
10	480	60	1,920	20,480
20	1,280	80	1,280	15,360

[1] Cultures were seeded with 6×10^6 mononuclear cells/ml isolated from plateletpheresis residues by Ficoll-Hypaque centrifugation. IFN yields were determined in culture fluids collected 48 to 72 h after the addition of OKT3-antibody.

Considerable variation was seen in the amount of IFN produced with cultures established from plateletpheresis residues from individual donors.

The yields of IFN obtained after stimulation with OKT3 were quite similar to the yields received on parallel stimulation with PHA [25]. Furthermore, OKT3-induced IFN production could be enhanced by co-stimulation with TPA or mezerein and the IFN thus produced had characteristics of IFN-γ. Thus, stimulation with commercially available OKT3 antibody represents an alternative means for human IFN-γ induction.

Some Characteristics of Human IFN-γ

IFN produced by combined stimulation with TPA and PHA showed characteristics most typically associated with IFN-γ: (a) the bulk of activity was destroyed on overnight dialysis at pH 2 and (b) its activity was neither neutralized nor bound by antisera raised against human IFN-α or IFN-β. A number of additional characteristics of this IFN were determined [19, 20], as summarized in table IV. These properties allow a clear differentiation between the IFN-γ and IFN-α or IFN-β species. Preliminary physicochemical characterization suggests that IFN-γ is structurally very markedly different from the other IFN species.

Table IV. Characteristics of human IFN-γ produced by combined stimulation with TPA and PHA

Treatment	Result
Dialysis at pH 2	≥ 80% inactivated
Anti-IFN-α or anti-IFN-β serum	No inactivation, no binding
Anti-IFN-γ serum	Neutralization
Chromatography on Con-A-Sepharose	Bound, eluted with α-D-mannopyranoside
Chromatography on controlled pore glass	Bound, eluted with ethylene glycol
Chromatography on Biogel P-100 or P-200	Apparent mol. weight 58,000 ± 3,000
Isoelectric focusing or chromatofocusing	Major component with pI 8.5
Sodium dodecyl sulfate, 0.1%	≥ 95% inactivated
β-Mercaptoethanol, 0.1 M	No inactivation
Incubation with bovine cells	No antiviral action detectable

Table V. Lack of correlation between titers of IFN-α, IFN-β and IFN-γ in different assay systems

Assay systems		Interferon titer[1]			Ratio of titers	
Cell	Virus	IFN-α	IFN-β	IFN-γ	α/γ	β/γ
FS7	VSV	128	128	< 16	> 8	> 8
	EMC	1,024	384	64	16	6
WISH	VSV	64	64	96	0.66	0.66
	EMC	256	256	1,024	0.25	0.25
A549	VSV	< 16	<16	< 16	–	–
	EMC	768	128	1,536	0.5	0.08

[1] IFN-α and IFN-β preparations used in these assays were diluted to contain 100 international units/ml. IFN-γ is an internal laboratory standard arbitrarily assigned a value of 256 "laboratory" units/ml.

In view of the marked physicochemical differences it is not surprising that the biological activities of IFN-γ are also quite different from the other human IFN species. Table V provides a summary of comparative titrations of human IFN-α, IFN-β, and IFN-γ preparations in three different cell lines challenged with two viruses. FS7 is a human diploid foreskin fibroblast strain routinely used in our laboratory; WISH is a line of transformed human amnion cells and A549 is a human lung carcinoma line. IFN titers were determined by assay in 96-well microplates after challenge with either vesicular stomatitis virus (VSV) or mouse encephalomyocarditis (EMC) virus, using 50% inhibition of cytopathic effect as the endpoint. The relative potency of IFN-γ was quite different from IFN-α or IFN-β in the different assay systems. IFN-γ was relatively less potent in FS7-cells but more active in WISH- and A549-cells. The resulting ratios of IFN-α/IFN-γ or IFN-β/IFN-γ titers calculated for the various cell-virus combinations could differ by as much as 100-fold. These results support the notion that the mechanism of IFN-γ action is significantly different from that of IFN-α or IFN-β.

Conclusions

There has been a rapid accumulation of new information about the structure and genetic organization of various IFNs. IFN-γ is clearly only now starting to catch up with its more fortunate relatives. However, an auspicious start has been made towards the goal of unraveling the nature and functions of the still enigmatic IFN-γ species.

It is likely that, as production methods are further improved, more IFN-γ will be available for laboratory research. This should lead to rapid further progress in the purification of this IFN and in the analysis of its molecular mechanisms of action.

In the meantime some progress is being made in the characterization of human IFN-γ mRNA [26, 27]. This work should ultimately lead to the cloning of complementary DNA, making possible rapid elucidation of the complete structure of IFN-γ. Cloning could also provide the ultimate means for the production of ample quantities of IFN-γ for clinical use.

Is the promise of IFN-γ as a potent, clinically useful immunoregulatory and antitumor agent likely to become a reality? The answer is, of course, not yet known. Those hoping to use this IFN as a magic bullet for cancer might find that reality will not have fully lived up to their expectations. As is the case with the other IFNs, IFN-γ is also not likely to be a panacea. But unraveling the mysteries of structure and function of this fascinating molecule is certainly an important enough challenge!

Acknowledgments

We thank *Michele Cassano, Angel Feliciano, Dorothy Henriksen Leela Jashnani,* and *Irene Zerebeckyj-Eckhardt* for technical assistance. This work was supported by U. S. Public Health Service Grants RO1-AI-07057, AI-12948, contract NO1-02169, and by grants from Flow Laboratories, Inc. and Rentschler Arzneimittel GmbH & Co.

References

1 Committee on Interferon Nomenclature: Interferon nomenclature. Nature *286:* 110 (1980).

2 Crane, J. L.; Glasgow, L. A.; Kern, E. R.; Youngner, J. S.: Inhibition of murine osteogenic sarcomas by treatment with type I or type II interferon. J. natn. Cancer. Inst. *61:* 871 – 874 (1978).

3 Rubin, B. Y.; Gupta, S. L.: Differential efficacies of human type I and type II interferons as antiviral and antiproliferative agents. Proc. natn. Acad. Sci. USA *77: 5928 – 5932* (1980).

4 Sonnenfeld, G.; Mandell, A.; Merigan, T. C.: Time and dosage dependence of immunoenhancement by murine type II interferon preparations. Cell. Immunol. *40:* 285 – 293 (1978).

5 Dianzani, T.; Salter, L.; Fleischman, R.; Zucca, M.: Immune interferon activates cells more slowly than does virus-induced interferon. Proc. Soc. exp. Biol. Med. *159:* 94 – 97 (1978).

6 Ankel, H.; Krishnamurti, C.; Besançon F.; Stefanos, S.; Falcoff, E.: Mouse fibroblast (type I) and immune (type II) interferons. Pronounced differences in affinity for gangliosides and in antiviral and antigrowth effects on mouse leukemia L-1210R cells. Proc. natn. Acad. Sci. USA *77:* 2528 – 2532 (1980).

7 Fleischmann, W. R.; Kleyn, K. M.; Baron, S.: Potentiation of antitumor effect of virus-induced interferon by mouse immune interferon preparations. J. natn. Cancer Inst. *65:* 963 – 966 (1980).

8 Wheelock, E. F.: Interferon-like virus-inhibitor induced in human leukocytes by phytohemagglutinin. Science *149:* 310 – 311 (1965).

9 De Ley, M.; Van Damme, J.; Claeys, H.; Weening, H.; Heine, J. W.; Billiau, A.; Vermylen, C.; De Somer, P.: Interferon induced in human leukocytes by mitogens: Production, partial purification, and characterization. Eur. J. Immunol. *10:* 877 – 883 (1980).

10 Langford, M. P.; Stanton, G. J.; Johnson, H. M.: Biological effects of staphylococcal enterotoxin-A on human peripheral lymphocytes. Infect. Immunity *22:* 62 – 68 (1978).

11 Falcoff, R.; Oriol, R.; Isacki, S.: Lymphocyte stimulation and interferon induction by 7S anti-human lymphocyte globulins and their uni and divalent fragments. Eur. J. Immunol. *2:* 476 – 478. (1972).

12 Dianzani, F.; Monahan, T. M.; Scupham, A.; Zucca, M.: Enzymatic induction of interferon production by galactose oxidase treatment of human lymphoid cells. Infect. Immunity *26:* 879 – 882 (1979).

13 Dianzani, F.; Monahan, T.; Georgiades, J.; Alperin, J. B.: Human immune interferon: Induction in lymphoid cells by a calcium ionophore. Infect. Immunity *29:* 561 – 563 (1980).

14 Ratliff, T. L.; McCool, R. E.; Catalona, W. J.: Interferon induction and augmentation of natural-killer activity by *Staphylococcus* protein-A. Cell. Immunol. *57:* 1 – 12 (1981).

15 Wang, J. L.; McClain, D. A.; Edelman, G. M.: Modulation of lymphocyte mitogenesis. Proc. natn. Acad. Sci. USA *72:* 1917 – 1921 (1975).

16 Mastro, A. M.; Mueller, G. C.: Synergistic action of phorbol esters in mitogen-activated bovine lymphocytes. Expl. Cell Res. *88:* 40 – 46 (1974).

17 Klein, G.; Vilček, J.: Attempts to induce interferon production by IUDR-induction and EBV-superinfection in human lymphoma lines and their hybrids. J. gen. Virol. *46:* 111 – 117 (1980).

18 Vilček, J.; Sulea, I. T.; Volvovitz, F.; Yip, Y. K.: Characteristics of interferons produced in cultures of human lymphocytes by stimulation with *Corynebacterium parvum* and phytohemagglutinin. In: Weck, Kristensen, Landy (eds.), Biochemical Characterization of Lymphokines, pp. 323 – 329 (Academic Press, New York 1980).

19 Yip, Y. K.; Pang, R. H. L.; Urban, C.; Vilček, J.: Partial purification and characterization of human gamma (immune) interferon. Proc. natn. Acad. Sci. USA *78:* 1601 – 1605 (1981).

20 Yip, Y. K.; Pang, R. H. L.; Oppenheim, J. D.; Nachbar, M. S.; Henriksen, D.; Zerebeckyj-Eckhardt, I.; Vilček, J.: Stimulation of human gamma (immune) interferon production by diterpene esters. Infect. Immunity (in press).

21 Mufson, R. A.; Fischer, S. M.; Verma, A. K.; Gleason, G. L.; Slaga, T. J.; Boutwell, R. K.: Effects of 12-0-tetradecanoylphorbol-13-acetate and mezerein on epidermal ornithine decarboxylase activity, isoproterenol-stimulated levels of cyclic adenosine 3':5'-monophosphate, and induction of mouse skin tumors in vivo. Cancer Res. *39:* 4791 – 4795 (1979).

22 Kaneko, Y.; Yatsuzuka, M.; Endo, Y.; Oda, T.: Activation of human lymphocytes by tumor promoter teleocidin. Biochem. biophys. Res. Commun. *100:* 888 – 893 (1981).

23 Van Wauwe, J. P.; De Mey, J. R.; Goossens, J. G.: OKT3: A monoclonal anti-human T-lymphocyte antibody with potent mitogenic properties. J. Immun. *124:* 2708 – 2713 (1980).

24 Kung, P. C.; Goldstein, G.; Reinherz, E. L.; Schlossman, S.: Monoclonal antibodies defining distinctive human T-cell surface antigens. Science *206:* 347 – 349 (1979).

25 Pang, R. H. L.; Yip, Y. K.; Vilček, J.: Immune interferon induction by a monoclonal antibody specific for human T-cells. Cell. Immunol. (in press).

26 Wallace, D. M.; Hitchcock, M. J. M.; Reber, S. B.; Berger, S. L.: Translation of human immune interferon messenger RNA in *Xenopus laevis* oocytes. Biochem. biophys. Res. Commun. *100:* 865 – 871 (1981).

27 Taniguchi, T.; Pang, R. H. L.; Yip, Y. K.; Henriksen, D.; Vilček, J.: Partial characterization of gamma (immune) interferon mRNA extracted from human lymphocytes. Proc. natn. Acad. Sci. USA *78:* 3469 – 3472 (1981).

Prof. J. Vilček, MD, New York University School of Medicine, 550 First Avenue, USA-NewYork, NY 10016

Clinical Trials of Human Leukocyte Interferon at the Memorial Sloan-Kettering Cancer Center

Herbert F. Oettgen und Susan E. Krown

Memorial Sloan-Kettering Cancer Center, New York, USA

At the Memorial Sloan-Kettering Cancer Center, we began to treat cancer patients with interferon in a systematic fashion in May 1979. We have treated patients with non-small-cell lung cancer, malignant melanoma, lymphomas, and osteogenic sarcoma in Phase-II trials aimed primarily at determining efficacy in these types of cancer. In a Phase-I trial examining the clinical pharmacology of interferon, we have treated patients with a variety of cancers. The total number of patients treated at Memorial Hospital is 82, the total number of patients treated in these trials 131 (table I). This number includes the patients treated at UCLA, Yale University, Stanford University, and M. D. Anderson Hospital in the two cooperative trials in melanoma and lymphoma. The interferon used in all trials was partially purified human leukocyte interferon prepared according to Cantell's method in laboratories at the Finnish Red Cross or the

Table I. Clinical trials of HuIFN-α (Le) at the Memorial Sloan-Kettering Cancer Center

Trial	No. of patients
Non-small-cell lung cancer	20
Malignant melanoma (with UCLA and Yale University)	17 (42*)
Lymphoma (with Stanford University and M. D. Anderson Hospital)	11 (35*)
Osteogenic sarcoma	8
Phase I	26
Total	82 (131)

* Total number of patients including those from other institutions

Kocher Institute in Berne. The specific activity of the preparations used was $0.5-1.0 \times 10^6$ U/mg protein. The new designation for this material is HuIFN-α (Le). With the exception of the Phase-I trial, the doses and schedules used were in part dictated by the limited availability of interferon.

Our first trial involved patients with non-small-cell carcinoma of the lung [1]. The aims of the trial were to assess the activity of leukocyte interferon in terms of tumor inhibition, toxicity, and effects on immune functions. The patients were treated at two dose levels, 3×10^6 U or 10×10^6 U/ day by i.m. injection for 30 days. Criteria of eligibility for this trial were a histologically confirmed diagnosis, measurable tumor outside previously irradiated fields, a performance status of more than 50%, adequate bone-marrow function, and no other therapy during the 4 weeks preceding the interferon trial.

20 patients were entered, 15 at the dose of 3×10^6 U and 5 at the dose of 10×10^6. 19 patients were evaluable, 17 with adenocarcinomas and 2 with epidermoid carcinomas. There were 9 men and 11 women, the median age was 50 years, and the performance status (Karnofsky scale) ranged from 60–90.

All patients except one had been treated before with other modalities, 11 with chemotherapy alone, 1 with radiation therapy alone, and 7 with radiation therapy and chemotherapy. 10 patients had shown objective tumor regression in response to these treatments – 8 showed a partial response, and 2 showed a minor response. All responses were induced with chemotherapy combinations that included cis-platinum, and all but 1 included vindesine as well. It should be noted that, as a general rule, patients, who have been treated extensively with chemotherapy or radiation therapy, are expected to respond less well to subsequent treatment with these modalities.

As some confusion exists regarding the meaning of the term "response", the criteria that we used are shown in table II. A decrease in the size of measurable lesions that qualifies as a response under the terms outlined in table II was not seen in any of the patients (table III). 11 patients showed stable disease during treatment and for at least 30 days thereafter. Progressive disease was seen in 8 patients. 1 patient noted improvement in rib pain, and showed disappearance of gynecomastia which recurred several weeks after treatment was stopped. Another patient showed some decrease in size of his lung tumor but no change in liver metastases.

Table II. Definition of response

Complete response (CR)	Disappearance of all detectable disease for 30 days
Partial response (PR)	Reduction of measurable lesions by at least 50% for 30 days
Minor response (MR)	Reduction of measurable lesions by at least 25% for 30 days
Stable disease (S)	Change of measurable lesions by less than 25% for 30 days
Progressive disease (P)	Increase of measurable lesions by at least 25% or appearance of new lesions

Table III. Results in patients with non-small-cell lung cancer

Result	Dose	
	3×10^6 U/day	10×10^6 U/day
Complete response	0	0
Partial response	0	0
Minor response	0	0
Stable disease	8/15	3/4
Progressive disease	7/15	1/4

Table IV. Clinical toxicity at the dose of 3×10^6 U/day

Type	No. of patients
Fever	
Mean peak 39.1°C	15/15
Range 38.1–40.3°C	
Chills	13/15
Fatigue, malaise, anorexia	14/15
Headache	5/15

Treatment with partially purified leukocyte interferon was not without side effects (table IV). All patients had fever on the first day of treatment, with a mean peak temperature of 39.1°C, and temperatures as high as 40.3°C. Half of the patients experienced shaking chills. Fever and chills generally did not recur after the first day or two of treatment. Headache was reported by one-third of the patients. The most disturbing subjective side effect developed during the second week of treatment. At that time, most patients experienced moderate or severe fatigue, general malaise, and anorexia, which limited

Table V. Hematologic toxicity

Type of blood cell	No. of patients	Results	
		Pre-treatment	Nadir
Leukocytes	14	8,300 ± 950*	4,000 ± 510
Granulocytes	14	6,116 ± 632	2,693 ± 439
Lymphocytes	14	1,424 ± 173	788 ± 100
Platelets	15	328,000 ± 38,000	197,000 ± 19,000

* Mean ± SE

normal activities in most cases. These symptoms eventually resolved, but not until 1 – 2 weeks after treatment was stopped.

All patients showed a decrease in total white blood cell count, absolute neutrophil count, and absolute lymphocyte count (table V). Once the nadir was reached, the count generally stabilized and, in some cases, even increased despite continued treatment. Bone-marrow hypoplasia was not seen. Only one patient showed a white blood cell count of less than 2500 and a granulocyte count of less than 1000. Moderate decreases in platelet count and hemoglobin concentration were also seen, but a platelet count of less than 100000 was found only in two patients who showed progressing bone-marrow metastases. Except in patients with bone-marrow involvement by tumor, the hematologic abnormalities were completely reversed 1 – 2 weeks after interferon was stopped.

A significant increase in the serum concentration of at least one liver enzyme was seen in 14 of 15 patients (table VI). Again these changes were rapidly reversible once treatment was stopped.

The trial in malignant melanoma sponsored by the American Cancer Society involves three institutions – UCLA and Yale University in addition to our own. Patients with skin, lymph-node or pulmonary metastases are eligible. They are stratified for having or not having lung metastases and then randomized to receive interferon at a dose of 1×10^6, 3×10^6, or 9×10^6 U by daily i.m. injection for 6 weeks. The trial has not yet been completed, and only preliminary results are available [2]. Of 43 evaluable patients, 21 had cutaneous or subcutaneous and/or lymph-node metastases only, and 22 had pulmonary metastases. 1 patient with cutaneous metastases only showed a partial response, and 2 patients with pulmonary metastases showed

Table VI. Liver enzymes

Enzyme	No. of patients	Result	
		Pre-treatment	Maximum
Alkaline phosphatase	15	119 ± 16.6*	203 ± 38.7
SGOT	15	34 ± 5.0	76 ± 19.7
γ-Glutamyl transpeptidase	14	57 ± 32.1	155 ± 64.3
5'Nucleotidase	14	11 ± 2.4	35 ± 9.2

* Mean ± SE

a minor response. 3 other patients with cutaneous or subcutaneous metastases showed evidence of therapeutic activity that did not qualify as a response under our accepted terms. 2 showed intense inflammation around metastatic lesions, associated in one patient with partial regression of 2 of 8 lesions. The third patient showed complete regression of 20 of 23 cutaneous lesions but developed 2 new subcutaneous metastases at the same time. 10 patients showed stable disease, 27 progressing disease. The responses occurred at all 3 dose levels. The side effects were the same as those seen in the lung-cancer trial.

Participants in the lymphoma trial, also sponsored by the American Cancer Society, have been the groups at Stanford University and the M. D. Anderson Hospital in addition to our group. Patients with nodular poorly differentiated lymphoma, nodular mixed lymphoma, diffuse well-differentiated lymphoma or chronic lymphocytic leukemia, diffuse histocytic lymphoma, or Hodgkin's disease are eligible. The design is similar to that of the melanoma trial in that the patients are randomized to receive a dose of 1×10^6, 3×10^6, or 9×10^6 U by daily i.m. injection. It differs from the melanoma trial in that the patients are treated for 4 weeks only. To date, 35 patients have been entered. It is much too early to estimate the frequency and duration of response for the various patient categories in this trial. One of our patients with nodular mixed lymphoma may serve as an example of a response. The patient had not been treated before with other modalities. He presented with generalized lymphadenopathy, splenomegaly, and bone-marrow involvement. Marked enlargement of iliac and paraaortic lymph nodes was seen in the lymphangiogram. After 2 weeks of treatment with interferon at the dose of 9×10^6 U/day, regression of palpable lymph nodes and spleen was observed, and re-

Table VII. Preliminary results in patients with malignant melanoma

Result	Total	Patients	
		No lung metastases	Lung metastases
Complete response	0	0	0
Partial response	1	1	0
Minor response	2	0	2
"Other" response	3	3	0
Stable disease	10	5	5
Progressive disease	27	12	15
Total evaluable	43	21	22

gression of lymph nodes was also seen in the lymphangiogram. At the end of the 4-week course of treatment, spleen and lymph nodes were no longer palpable but the bone marrow still contained lymphoma cells. Four weeks later (without further treatment), the bone marrow was found to be normal. The patient remained in complete remission for 10 months without any treatment. When relapse occurred, a second complete response was induced with interferon. The patient is still in complete remission.

Our trial in patients with osteogenic sarcoma started only a few months ago. Patients with recurrent or metastatic tumor are eligible if their performance status and bone-marrow function are adequate, and if they have had no other treatment for four weeks. The patients are first treated at a dose of 3×10^6 U/day given by i.m. injection for 30 days, and this is followed by a 4-week course of treatment at a daily dose of 10×10^6 U. At this early stage of the trial, only 8 patients can be evaluated. While 4 patients showed a decrease in elevated alkaline phosphatase levels (generally considered a sensitive parameter of disease activity), a measurable decrease in tumor size has not yet been observed.

The last trial of our current series is a Phase-I trial. In contrast to other new agents in cancer therapy, interferon has not had Phase-I trials during the earliest phase of clinical application – in part because it was considered non-toxic, and in part because the shortage of supply forced priorities in the direction of establishing efficacy in the treatment of tumors that appeared most susceptible initially to inhibition by interferon. The aims of our current Phase-I trial at Memorial Hospital are to determine the maximum tolerated dose and toxicity of

Table VIII. Phase-I trial of HuIFN-α (Le)

Diagnosis	No. of patients treated	No. of patients showing an antitumor effect
Breast cancer	7	1
Colon cancer	4	
Malignant melanoma	4	1
Lymphoma	7	3 (1 CR, 2 PR)
Ovarian cancer	1	
Multiple myeloma	1	
Adenocarcinoma, ? primary	1	

leukocyte interferon given at a single dose or on daily schedules, and to define the effects of different doses and schedules on immune functions, pharmacokinetics, and tumor growth. The trial is far from complete.

To date, 26 patients with 10 different types of advanced cancers have been entered (table VIII). So far, the patients have received doses of 1, 2.5, 5, 10, and 15×10^6 U i.m. as single doses or by daily injection for up to 60 days. Because of unacceptable toxicity, it has not yet been possible to give the dose of 15×10^6 U on a daily schedule. 5 of the 26 patients showed evidence of an antitumor effect. The patient with subcutaneous chest wall metastases of breast cancer, had been treated extensively with chemotherapy and radiation therapy in the past. Because of marked orthostatic hypotension, the daily dose of interferon had to be reduced from 10×10^6 U to 2.5×10^6 U. The patient showed regression of chest wall lesions by 50% for two weeks, followed by progression despite continued treatment. The patient with malignant melanoma had multiple subcutaneous metastases, previously treated without much success with MER, BCG, and DTIC. During treatment with interferon, the skin metastases showed some decrease in size but eventually progressed again. This patient is the only patient we have seen who developed generalized urticaria in association with the interferon injections. They were easily controlled with antihistamines.

Three patients in the lymphoma group showed evidence of antitumor activity that qualifies as a complete [1] or partial [2] response. The first patient, with nodular mixed lymphoma, is the patient described earlier as having shown a complete response to treatment at 9×10^6 U for 30 days. When he relapsed 10 months later with general-

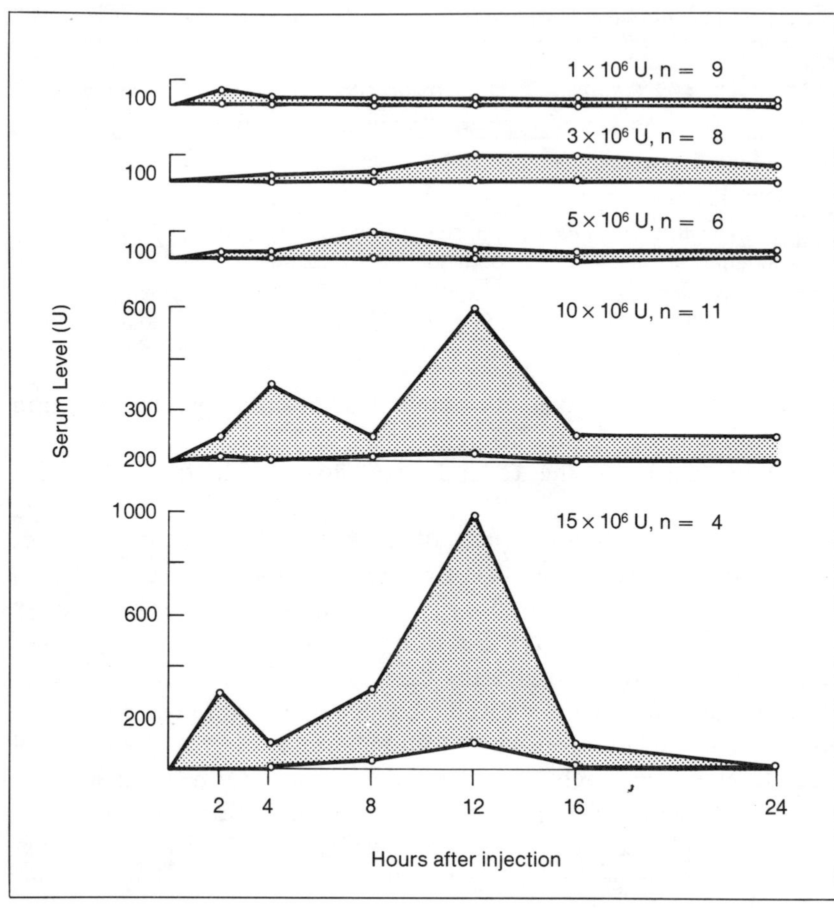

Figure 1. Serum levels of interferon after i. m. injection of HuIFN-α (Le).

ized lymphadenopathy, splenomegaly, and bone-marrow involvement, he was treated at the dose of 5×10^6 U/day for 8 weeks and achieved again complete remission after 4 weeks of treatment. The second patient, with partially nodular and partially diffuse mixed lymphoma, presented with extensive lymphadenopathy and patchy bone-marrow involvement. He had not been treated before and has so far shown a partial response after one month of treatment at the dose of 5×10^6 U/day. Treatment is being continued. The third patient, with mycosis fungoides, showed complete regression of extensive skin lesions in response to interferon treatment at the dose of

Table IX. Effects of HuIFN-α (Le) on the proliferative response of peripheral blood lymphocytes to phytohemagglutinins

Time of test	No. of patients	Result (mean CPM ± SEM)
Before treatment	12	15,096 ± 1,255
After treatment		
Day 1 – 2	12	13,654 ± 1,152
Week 1	12	12,626 ± 1,461
Week 2	11	11,842 ± 1,472
Week 3 – 4	11	9,662 ± 1,958

Table X. Effects of HuIFN-α (Le) on the proliferative response of peripheral blood lymphocytes to antigens

Antigen	No. of patients	Result (mean CPM ± SEM)		
		Before	After (24 h)	% Decrease
C. albicans	19	8,023 ± 1,237	3,486 ± 701	57
E. coli	15	2,013 ± 513	624 ± 218	69
S. aureus	14	3,194 ± 786	898 ± 303	72
PPD	19	3,710 ± 998	1,871 ± 736	50

5×10^6 U/day. While the skin lesions regressed completely, enlarged lymph nodes decreased only very slightly in size and began to enlarge rapidly when interferon was discontinued.

Serum levels of interferon were measured in all of our clinical trials by a cytophatic effect inhibition assay on VSV-infected human fibroblasts. Individual variation of interferon levels has been considerable at all dose levels. Figure 1 illustrates the serum levels seen in 38 patients treated at a dose of 1, 3, 5, 10, or 15×10^6 U. The shaded areas represent the range of interferon levels. Levels are shown at 2, 4, 8, 12, 16, and 24 h after injection. At the dose of 15×10^6, for example, the peak level at 12 h was 1000 U/ml in one patient and only 100 U in another.

Let us now turn to some of the immunological changes seen in our patients. Interferon appears to inhibit the proliferative response of peripheral blood lymphocytes to a variety of stimuli. One example, the response to phytohemagglutinin, is shown in table IX. A gradual decline in the mean peak response to PHA was observed which became significant only after 3 – 4 weeks of treatment.

By contrast, the lymphoproliferative response to specific antigens

Table XI. Effects of HuIFN-α (Le) on natural-killer cell activity against K-562 target cells

Patient	Before treatment	Result (% specific ^{51}Cr release)		
		After treatment (days)		
		1–3	7	14–28
1	17	70	57	30
2	26	80	56	46
3	39	–	78	–
4	8	18	51	22
5	48	84	–	–
6	14	17	36	1
7	15	18	–	36
8	5	84	51	49
9	68	61	47	–
10	41	76	30	34
11	47	47	68	53
12	36	39	47	52
13	43	79	53	68

decreased immediately after the first dose of interferon. Table X summarizes results seen in tests with C. albicans, E. coli, S. S. aureus, and PPD one day after the first injection of 3×10^6 U, showing a 50–70% decrease of thymidine incorporation. The results were similar in patients treated at a dose of 1×10^6 U or 10×10^6 U.

One function of lymphocytes that has received much attention in interferon trials is the so-called natural-killer cell activity or spontaneous cell-mediated cytotoxicity. Table XI shows results obtained in patients treated at a dose of 3×10^6 U/day for 4 weeks in assays measuring NK activity of peripheral blood lymphocytes against K-562 target cells. Almost all patients who were tested within one week of starting treatment showed a significant increase – more than 50% over the pretreatment value – and in some cases the increase was sustained throughout treatment. Normal controls generally showed no more than 15–20% fluctuation with time, with a mean specific release of about 35% and a lower limit of about 20%. In this group of patients, no correlation between NK activity and serum levels of interferon was observed.

When we compare NK activity in patients treated at different dose levels, it appears that higher doses do not cause a greater increase. In a small series of 21 patients treated at 5 dose levels ranging from 1 to 15×10^6 U, the most regular and substantial increase of NK

Table XII. Changes in natural-killer cell activity against K-562 target cells after single doses of HuIFN-α (Le)

Dose (10^{-6} U IM)	Maximum increase (%) of specific ^{51}Cr release in individual patients	No. patients with > 50% increase/ No. patients tested
1.0	18, 170, 300	2/3
2.5	88, 221, 230	3/3
5.0	85, 196, 267, 276, 1,800	5/5
10.0	0, 0, 31, 66, 114, 159	3/6
15.0	0, 36, 94, 130	2/4

Table XIII. Cell-surface markers of peripheral blood mononuclear cells

Marker	Cells expressing the marker					
	Pre-B cells	B cells	Pre-T cells	T cells	Third population	Monocytes
Membrane Ig	–	+	–	–	–	± (IgG)
EAC rosette	–	+	±	–	+	+
Fc receptor						
EA (Ripley rosette)	–	–	–	–	+	±
Agg. IgG	–	+	–	–	±	+
Tμ, Tγ	–	–	–	+	–	–
Mouse rosette	–	+	–	–	–	–
SRBC rosette	–	–	–	+	–	–
Phagocytosis	–	–	–	–	–	+
Cytoplasmic IgM	+	–	–	–	–	–
Terminal transferase	±	–	+	–	–	–
"Ia-like" antigens	+	+	+	–	?	+

activity was seen in patients treated at intermediate dose levels (table XII). While these results are obviously preliminary, they remind us of the fact that the dose-response curve needs to be defined for each of the many parameters of interferon action, and that it may be biphasic for some parameters.

In addition to testing for changes in lymphocyte function, we have attempted to determine whether treatment with HuIFN-α (Le) induces changes in lymphocyte phenotype. A comprehensive analysis of lymphocyte surface markers (table XIII, XIV) has not shown consistent changes in the subpopulations identified by any single marker, including some of the markers defined by monoclonal antibodies. Recently, we have begun to examine effects of interferon on macrophage function. In one type of assay, we determined the release of interleukin-1 (IL-1) by the patients' peripheral blood monocytes in re-

Table XIV. T-cell subsets defined by monoclonal antibodies

Antibody	% Positive cells				Assigned function
	Thymo-cytes	Blood lympho-cytes	E + cells	Spleen cells	
leu 1	100	70	80–95		
leu 2a		20	25–45		Suppressor
leu 3a		50	45–75		Helper
leu 4		70	80–95		
OKT 3	20		100	30	
OKT 4	75		65	15	Helper
OKT 8	80		35	15	Suppressor

sponse to endotoxin in vitro. IL-1 has been shown to play a central role in the development of B-cell and T-cell precursors to functioning effector cells. It provides the signal that induces maturation of antigen-activated precursors to the point where they can respond to the proliferative signals that induce clonal expansion. IL-1 release by monocytes, normally triggered by a T-cell signal, can also be induced by endotoxin. When human monocytes are incubated with interferon rather than endotoxin, they also release IL-1. Initial tests indicate that this response may also occur in vivo when patients are treated with interferon.

As early as one day after the beginning of interferon treatment, the release of interleukin-1 by peripheral blood monocytes in response to endotoxin was found to be decreased (table XV), suggesting that the monocytes were stimulated by interferon to release interleukin-1 in vivo, and were consequently less responsive to endotoxin stimulation in vitro.

In another type of assay we can dissect the complex process of antibody production by human peripheral blood mononuclear cells in vitro, using a culture system that is similar to the Mishell-Dutton system used widely in studies of the regulation of antibody production in the mouse. Table XVI shows the results of tests in 5 patients before and after treatment with interferon. The patients' cells were sensitized in vitro with sheep red blood cells, and the number of antibody-secreting cells was determined several days later in a plaque assay. To determine effects of suppressor cells, the mononuclear cells were examined as an unfractionated population as well as after remo-

Table XV. Effects of treatment with HuIFN-α (Le) on the release of interleukin-1 by blood monocytes in response to endotoxin

Patient	Release of IL-1 (% of control) by monocytes in vitro in response to endotoxin	
	Before HuIFN-α (Le)	1 day after 3×10^6 U IM
1	140	75
2	73	6
3	42	7
4	66	19
5	212	13

Table XVI. Effects of treatment with HuIFN-α (Le) on in vitro antibody production by blood cells

Patient	Anti-SRBC PFC			
	Unfractionated PBL		Fractionated PBL*	
	Before treatment	After treatment	Before treatment	After treatment
1	0	0	0	263
2	0	0	0	2400
3	0	0	30	250
4	0	0	216	410
5	34	28	1900	1480

* Depleted of Sephadex G-10-adherent cells

val of Sephadex G-10-adherent cells. It appears that interferon treatment caused an increase in the number of antibody-secreting cells that became detectable when G-10-adherent cells were removed in those patients where antibody production before treatment was undetectable or minimal. Obviously, these observations made in only few patients are quite preliminary. Nevertheless, they provide hints at immunological effects of interferon that justify further investigation.

What can we conclude from these studies? First, it is clear that partially purified human leukocyte interferon can induce complete or partial regression of some types of human cancer in some patients. Second, it is equally clear that clinically useful responses have been quite rare in our experience, a statement which means little as long as we talk about patients who have been treated with highly impure interferon preparations at doses, and for periods of time, that were limited by availability more than anything else. Third, partially purified leukocyte interferon has its characteristic toxicity which is limiting at higher dose levels. Fourth, partially purified leukocyte interferon has profound immunological effects that offer intriguing opportunities for study. In assessing the therapeutic potential of interferons, we have barely begun to scratch the surface. What is fascinating is the fact that interferons have any effect at all on cancer. Now that highly purified interferons are becoming available in larger quantities from various sources, there is every reason to continue to define these effects and the mechanisms involved.

Acknowledgment

Participants in the studies discussed here were the following clinical investigators: *R. J. Gralla, M. Stoopler* (lung cancer), *C. Pinsky, D. Kerr, J. Kirkwood, J. Nordlund, M. Burk, D. Morton* (malignant melanoma), the group conducting the ACS lymphoma trial (*T. Merigan*, Chairman), *G. Rosen, B. Caparros* (osteogenic sarcoma), *T. Khansur, F. Real* (Phase I). Participating laboratory investigators were *W. E. Stewart, M. Krim, S. Cunningham-Rundles, B. Koziner* and *M. Hoffmann*. The studies were supported by grants from the National Cancer Institute (CA 08748 and CA 19267) and from the American Cancer Society.

References

1 Krown, S. E.; Stoopler, M. B.; Cunningham-Rundles, S.; Oettgen, H. F.: Phase-II trial of human leukocyte interferon (IFN) in non-small-cell lung cancer (NSCLC). Proc. Am. Assoc. Cancer Res. *21:* 179 (1980).

2 Krown, S. E.; Burk, M.; Kirkwood, J. M.; Kerr, D.; Nordlund, J. J.; Morton, D. L.; Oettgen, H. F.: Human leukocyte interferon (HuLeIF) in malignant melanoma (MM): Preliminary report of the American Cancer Society clinical trial. Proc. Am. Assoc. Cancer Res. *22:* 158 (1981).

H. F. Oettgen, MD, Memorial Sloan-Kettering Cancer Center, 1275 York Avenue, USA- New York, N.Y. 10021

Perspectives for Clinical Use of Fibroblast Interferon

P. De Somer

Rega Institute, University of Leuven, Belgium

Introduction

Leukocyte interferon has been available for clinical experiments for several years. Fibroblast interferon, in contrast, has only recently been prepared in sufficient amounts to test its effect after systemic administration in man. As a result of this, little published information is as yet available [3, 6, 11, 17, 27, 28, 31, 39, 40]. In the past five years relatively large quantities of fibroblast interferon have been produced at the Rega Institute by the classical method of superinduction in diploid skin fibroblasts. It was purified by adsorption to controlled pore glass at neutral pH and desorption by acid [2, 4]. This interferon has been given to about 47 patients with various pathologies in an attempt to test tolerability and pharmacokinetics, and to define viral or other diseases that may favorably respond to fibroblast interferon therapy [3, 5, 6, 17, 39, 40].

Fibroblast Interferon Therapy in Viral Diseases

Our strategy for designing clinical experiments was based on the observation in animal studies that interferon fails to protect against viral diseases if given at the time when clinical symptoms are already apparent [13, 14, 15, 19, 21, 25]. Also, on merely theoretical grounds, the use of interferon has little chance to be effective during the acute phase of viral disease. Indeed, viral invasion of a particular organ is accompanied by the local production of large amounts of endogenous interferon [25, 26, 38]. From this it may be postulated that, for exogenous interferon to exert a favorable effect, it should reach the sites of viral involvement either earlier or in much higher concentrations than the endogenous interferon produced by the viral infection itself.

For this reason it was decided to select diseases that could be treated prophylactically (e. g. patients who are particularly exposed to viral infections) and diseases caused by virus infections that induce little or no endogenous interferon (e.g. chronic infections). A summary of these trials, performed with fibroblast interferon and prepared at our institute, is given in table I.

The prophylactic effect of systemic interferon treatment on viral infections was tested in a placebo-controlled trial on renal transplant patients. As these patients are highly susceptible to viral infections, it was anticipated that meaningful results would be obtained from a small number of patients treated. 8 patients received 3 MU of fibroblast interferon twice weekly for 6 weeks, starting on the day of transplantation. No statistically significant effect was seen on the general incidence or severity of viral infections. There was only a suggestive decrease in the severity of herpes simplex virus. In similar experiments with leukocyte interferon, a reduction in cytomegalovirus shedding was seen [12]. However, this reduction was not accompanied by a dramatical clinical benefit for treated as opposed to non-treated patients.

In some viral infections the endogenous production of interferon is minimal or non-existent, thereby increasing the chances for exogenous interferon to affect the course of the disease. As a therapeutic model hepatitis-B was chosen, because, unlike in other viral infections, there are stable levels of viral proteins, which can be measured in liver and blood, i.e. HBc antigen, HBs antigen, HBe antigen, and DNA polymerase. Thus, a treatment insufficient to cause clinical benefit might, nevertheless, reveal the presence of an antiviral action.

Three patients, hospitalized for moderately severe acute hepatitis-B, were treated with daily i.m. injections of 2 MU for 2 weeks. No striking effect on the evolution of these cases of moderate intensity was observed. In fact, no features distinguishing these cases from untreated cases were noticed, except for a somewhat prolonged presence of HBs antigen in the serum.

Table I. Overview of clinical trials on viral diseases conducted with fibroblast interferon prepared at the Rega Institute

Disease	No. of patients	No. of injections given	Dose of interferon (MU/injection)	Duration of treatment (days)	Evaluation of effect	References
Acute hepatitis-B	3	14	2.0	14	Recovery as expected; HBsAg positive for 2 to 3 months	3, 6
Fulminant hepatitis-B	4	5–10	3.5–6.0	5–15	Two patients died (day 5–7); two recovered	3, 6
Papilloma of larynx	3	13–40	3–4	18–90	Partial regression	3, 6, 34
Common warts	3	8–14	3.5–5.9	14–24	Regression of small warts in 1 patient (renal transplant); not in 2 others	3, 6
Condyloma accuminatum	2	8	3.5	14	Stationary	3, 6
Chronic hepatitis-B	9	7–28	0.1–10	7–28	Permanent improvement in 3 patients; transient improvement in 3 patients; unaltered disease in 3 patients	3, 6, 40
Prophylaxis of virus infection in renal transplant patients (placebo-controlled)	8	26	3.0	42	Suggestive of effect on incidence of herpes-I	3, 39

Fulminant hepatitis was chosen as another indication because it was reasoned that interferon, by quickly lowering the virus load, could tip the balance from death to life, at least in those cases in which the liver was not irreversibly damaged. 4 patients were treated with 3.5 MU daily for 5 days, followed by 5 additional doses every 2 days. 2 patients survived, 2 of them died within a few days after initiation of treatment.

Fibroblast interferon was also given to 9 patients with chronic active hepatitis-B for time periods ranging from 2 to 5 weeks. Out of these 9 patients, 3 showed a permanent improvement in viral as well as clinical parameters, 4 patients showed transient and/or ambiguous responses, 2 patients failed to respond. The interpretation of these results is complicated by the fact that little is known about the natural history of chronic active hepatitis: the favorable evolution seen in some of the patients may have been spontaneous rather than provoked by interferon. Even if the improvement could be related to the administration of interferon, the possibility remains that the favorable effects were due to the pharmacological activity of impurities in the interferon preparation. In view of these difficulties we decided to postpone a controlled study until the administration of higher doses and of pure interferon becomes feasible. It was felt that the benefit, observed in the pilot trials, was too small and too uncertain to justify a major financial effort.

Six cases of chronic infection with papilloma virus (cutaneous, laryngeal, or venereal) were treated with i.m. injections of 3.5 – 5.9 MU/day daily or every other day for 1 – 3 weeks. We were encouraged by the regression of small verrucae planae in a renal transplant carrier with multiple cutaneous warts. *Schouten and Bos* [34] used fibroblast interferon from our laboratory to treat 2 patients with laryngeal papilloma (subcutaneous injections of 4 MU, 3 times weekly, for 3 months), and reported regression during treatment followed by recurrence after discontinuation of treatment. A suggestive beneficial effect (partial rejection of the papilloma) was also seen in a third patient given a short course of fibroblast interferon treatment [3, 6]. No changes were seen in the other patients.

In some, but not all, patients, fibroblast interferon evoked febrile reactions, delayed skin reactivity, and transient lymphopenia. Some patients developed an allergic state of the reaginic type as evidenced by a wheel and flare reaction after intradermal challenge. Evidence was obtained indicating that these side effects were due to impurities [8].

The purpose of the pilot trials that we have performed was to provide a basis for the selection of certain diseases that might be suitable targets for fibroblast interferon therapy. Furthermore, the results of these pilot trials were to guide us in selecting dosage schedules. The conclusions that we have reached were such that we decided not to give priority to further clinical trials on viral diseases. This conclusion was justified by the fact that, with the current dosage schedules:

(1) no spectacular cures occurred in acute virus diseases, exemplified by acute hepatitis-B;
(2) there was no clear-cut prophylactic effect on the occurrence of acute viral diseases in high-risk patients;
(3) in chronic viral diseases, exemplified by chronic hepatitis-B or viral papillomatosis, there was an indication that sustained treatment at high doses might result in clinical benefit. However, to achieve this would require the availability of fibroblast interferon preparations of higher purity and at lower costs.

Although the number of trials done with fibroblast interferon is smaller than that performed with leukocyte interferon, it is not our impression that the results in terms of clinical benefit are worse, or less certain. In fact, the trials conducted with leukocyte interferon are subject to the same type of criticism as those reported here for fibroblast interferon [7]. It is our feeling that further clinical trials should make use of pure interferon, either leukocyte or fibroblast, in order to establish that whatever beneficial effect was seen in the pilot trials was due to interferon and not to complex pharmacological activities.

Fibroblast Interferon Therapy in Cancer Patients

Current attempts to exploit interferons as antitumor agents stem from the observation that systemic administration of interferon can delay progression of experimentally induced tumors in mice [22]. The mechanism of this antitumor effect is believed to be multifactorial: inhibition of cell division, enhanced expression of membrane antigens, and activation of macrophages, sensitized T-lymphocytes, antibody-dependent cytotoxic lymphocytes, and lymphocytes with natural-killer activity [22].

Our research group became only reluctantly involved in clinical trials on tumor patients. We were particularly concerned by the high doses of interferon required in experiments on mice in order to obtain only modest effects, i.e. delay in outgrowth of the tumor. For instance, in order to delay the outgrowth of B16-melanoma or the occurrence of metastases of Lewis-lung carcinoma in mice, a daily dose of ~ 20 MU/kg was required [20]. Regression of experimental tumors such as that obtained with clinically successful chemotherapeutics (e.g. cyclophosphamide, melphalan, and the vinca alkaloids) have, with a single exception [29], never been reported in mice treated with interferon. For these reasons we had little hope to achieve clear-cut clinical benefit by treating patients with currently feasible doses (max. 30 MU/patient/day = 0.5 MU/kg/day). Our strategy was to conduct pilot trials on small numbers of patients in order to define the most likely candidate for interferon therapy.

Table II gives an overview of the tumor patients who, up to this date, have received fibroblast interferon from the production unit of our institute. Clear-cut progression of disease during treatment was seen in the patients with osteosarcoma, neuroblastoma, epithelioma of head and neck region, as well as in 2 of the 3 patients with light-chain myeloma. One of these 3 patients subsequently showed a favorable response to treatment with leukocyte interferon. One patient with a well-documented primary nasopharyngeal carcinoma, due to Epstein-Barr virus infection, received fibroblast interferon for 6 weeks prior to irradiation. Lymph nodes as well as the primary tumor in the pharynx were undetectable at the end of the interferon treatment course. However, the interpretation of the findings was obscured by the fact that extensive biopsies had been taken in the area of the primary tumor and that the lymph-node regression may in fact have been due to decrease in the inflammatory response. In a pilot trial on 3 patients with advanced, therapy-resistant breast cancer, regression of small metastatic nodules was observed in all 3 patients, followed by recurrence after treatment was discontinued. Large metastatic lesions were not responsive. This observation is by far the most encouraging that has been obtained with fibroblast interferon from our institute. It undoubtedly warrants further investigation of the interferon effects in breast cancer.

The number of tumor patients treated with fibroblast interferon is still too small to allow a conclusion as to which direction further trials should take. Nasopharyngeal carcinoma, in view of the experience of *Treuner et al.* [36] and ourselves, seems to be one possible candidate. It should be noted, however, that this tumor, which occurs primarily in Asia, can effectively be treated by radiotherapy. Another candidate seems to be breast cancer.

In West Germany (see the other presentations in this symposium) and in Japan [33], a large number of tumor patients are currently re-

Table II. Overview of clinical trials conducted on tumor patients using fibroblast interferon prepared at the Rega Institute

Disease	No. of patients	No of injections given	Dose of interferon (MU/injection)	Duration of treatment (days)	Evaluation of effect	References
Metastatic osteosarcoma (resistant to chemotherapy)	2	15–42	3.5	15–90[1]	Progressive disease	3, 6
Neuroblastoma[2]	1	18	1.7	28	Progressive disease	3, 6
Myeloma (light-chain disease)	3	14–75	3–10	30–132	Stable disease in 1 patient; progressive disease in 2 patients	10
Metastatic skin epithelioma (head and neck)	5	16	7	28	Progressive disease	Trial in progress (Prof. Dr. M. Vanderschueren, Academic Hospital, University of Leuven, Belgium)
Metastatic breast cancer	3	8	7	42	Regression of some small metastatic nodules; progression of cancer lesions	Trial in progress (Prof. Dr. P. Pouillart, Institut Curie, Paris, France)
Nasopharyngeal carcinoma	1	24	7	42	Apparent regression of primary tumor and lymph-node metastasis	(Prof. Dr. R. Verwilghen, Academic Hospital, University of Leuven, Belgium)

[1] 13 year old boy; [2] 3 year old girl.

ceiving fibroblast interferon. In these trials the interferon is mostly given by the i.v. route, as opposed to the i.m. route used in our experiments as well as in trials using leukocyte interferon. The reason for this choice was the observation, originally made in our laboratory [18], that blood titers of interferon in patients receiving i.m. injections of fibroblast interferon were much lower than those in patients receiving intramuscularly injected leukocyte interferon. Subsequent to this observation we have compared the pharmacokinetics of leukocyte and fibroblast interferon in various animal species [9]. Higher blood titers with leukocyte than with fibroblast interferon were found in rabbits injected intramuscularly and in mice injected intraperitoneally. In rhesus monkeys no difference was seen. Furthermore, in mice the interferon levels in tissues (lungs and spleen) were as high with fibroblast as with leukocyte interferon, despite a large difference in serum levels. This suggested that fibroblast interferon is removed rapidly from the circulation to become fixed in certain tissues.

Along the same line *Lucero et al.* [30], working with fibroblast interferon from our institute, found that i.m. injection of fibroblast and leukocyte interferon in patients resulted in equally pronounced activation of natural-killer activity of their peripheral blood mononuclear cells. Thus it seems that intramuscularly injected fibroblast interferon does reach certain internal organs as effectively as leukocyte interferon. We can see no reason to give preference to the i.v. administration route. In fact, side-effects, such as pyrexia, seem to be more pronounced and the risks to provoke acute allergic reactions may be higher.

Whereas it is still unclear which type of disease should be selected for further clinical trials, and which dosage schedule and administration routes should be preferred, it is sufficiently clear that a large effort should now be devoted to use purer preparations of fibroblast interferon. The reasons for this are obvious. In currently used preparations only 0.1 to 1% of the protein molecules present are interferon. Among the impurities are various pharmacologically active substances which one might refer to as cytokines. These are probably responsible for the so-called side-effects of therapy with fibroblast interferon: pyrexia, transient lymphopenia, local mononuclear cell infiltration in injected tissues [3, 5, 6, 16]. Extensive purification seems to remove these activities effectively [8]. Also some impure preparations seem to contain less of these substances than others. Thus, pyrexia is common in patients receiving fibroblast interferon prepared from diploid cells and is virtually absent when fibroblast interferon from the MG-63 cells is used (our unpublished results).

The goal of working with highly pure fibroblast interferon is now attainable by the existence of simple methods for complete purification [23, 24]. However, new complexities are arising by the apparent existence of subtypes of interferon molecules. In the case of leukocyte interferon, it is already well established that multiple genes exist, which code for similar but not identical HuIFN-α molecules [1, 32]. In the case of fibroblast interferon, evidence for the existence of multiple genes and their corresponding gene products is still controversial [35]. We have found that fibroblast interferon prepared from MG-63 cells contains 2 variants of HuIFN-β differing from each other in elution patterns from Zn-chelate columns [23, 24]. We also found that interferon preparations obtained by exposure of human peripheral blood mononuclear cells to concanavalin-A contain predominantly HuIFN-γ (immune type or type-II interferon) but also HuIFN-β and HuIFN-α. The HuIFN-β component was found to be different from classical HuIFN-β in its various biochemical and biological properties [37]. Therefore, in all likelihood, the coming months and years of interferon research will be marked by more complexity than the clinician would like to be confronted with.

A definitive conclusion regarding the clinical applicability of fibroblast interferon would be premature at this time. In fact, the question remains controversial for both interferons: the hope for a spectacular cancer cure has not materialized with either of the two interferons and there are only a few cases where interferon therapy seems to yield better results than conventional forms of therapy. The use of much higher doses or the combination of interferon with other forms of therapy could bring some change in this rather pessimistic picture. Meanwhile, interferons remain in the stage of "potent drugs in search of a disease".

Acknowledgment

The production of fibroblast interferon in the Rega Institute was largely made possible by grants received from the Cancer Research Foundation of the Belgian ASLK/CGER (General Savings and Retirement Fund) and from the Belgian Ministries of the Economy and of the Science Policy.

References

1 Allen, G.; Fantes, K. H.: A family of structural genes for human lymphoblastoid (leukocyte type) interferon. Nature *287:* 408–411 (1980).

2 Billiau, A.; Joniau, M.; De Somer, P.: Mass production of human interferon in diploid cells stimulated by poly-I: C. J. gen. Virol. *19:* 1–8 (1973).

3 Billiau, A.; Edy, V. G.; De Somer, P.: The clinical use of fibroblast interferon. In:

Chandra, Antiviral Mechanisms in the Control of Neoplasia, pp. 675–696 (Plenum Press, New York and London 1979).

4 Billiau, A.; Van Damme, J.; Van Leuven, F.; Edy, V. G.; De Ley, M.; Cassiman, J. J.; Van den Berghe, H.; De Somer, P.: Human fibroblast interferon for clinical trials: Production, partial purification, and characterization. Antimicrob. Agents Chemother. *16:* 49–55 (1979).

5 Billiau, A.; De Somer, P.; Edy, V. G.; De Clercq, E.; Heremans, H.: Human fibroblast interferon for clinical trials: Pharmacokinetics and tolerability in experimental animals and humans. Antimicrob. Agents Chemother. *16:* 56–63 (1979).

6 Billiau, A.; De Somer, P.: Clinical use of interferons in viral infections. In: Stringfellow, Interferon and Interferon Inducers, Clinical Applications, pp. 113–144 (Marcel Dekker Inc., New York and Basel 1980).

7 Billiau, A.; De Somer, P.; Schellekens, H.; Weimar, W.: The clinical value of interferon: A more critical appraisal. Neth. J. Med. (in press, 1980).

8 Billiau, A.; Heine, J. W.; Van Damme, J.; Heremans, H.; De Somer, P.: Tolerability of pure fibroblast interferon in man. Ann. N. Y. Acad. Sci. *350:* 374–375 (1980).

9 Billiau, A.: Interferon therapy: Pharmacokinetic und pharmacological aspects. Arch. Virol. *67:* 121–133 (1981).

10 Billiau, A.; Bloemmen, J.; Bogaerts, M.; Claeys, H.; Van Damme, J.; De Ley, M.; De Somer, P.; Drochmans, A.; Heremans, H.; Kriel, A.; Schetz, J.; Tricot, G.; Vermylen, C.; Verwilghen, R.; Waer, M.: Interferon therapy in myeloma failure of human fibroblast interferon administration to affect the course of light-chain disease. Eur. J. Cancer (submitted, 1981).

11 Carter, W. A.; Leong, S. S.; Horoszewicz, J. S.: Human fibroblast interferon in the control of neoplasia. In: Chandra, Antiviral Mechanisms in the Control of Neoplasia, pp. 663–674 (Plenum Press, New York and London 1979).

12 Cheeseman, S. H.; Rubin, R. H.; Stewart, J. A.; Tolkoff-Rubin, N. E.; Cosimi, A. B.; Cantell, K.; Gilbert, J.; Winkle, S.; Herrin, J. T.; Black, P. H.; Russell, P. S.; Hirsch, M. S.; Controlled clinical trial of prophylactic human leukocyte interferon in renal transplantation. New Engl. J. Med. *300:* 1345–1349 (1979).

13 De Clercq, E.; De Somer, P.: Protective effect of interferon and polyacrylic acid in newborn mice infected with a lethal dose of vesicular stomatitis virus. Life Sci. *7:* 925–933 (1968).

14 De Clercq, E.; De Somer, P.: Effect of interferon, polyacrylic acid, and polymethacrylic acid on tail lesions in mice infected with vaccinia virus. Appl. Microbiol. *16:* 1314–1319 (1968).

15 De Clercq, E.; De Somer, P.: Comparative study of the efficacy of different forms of interferon therapy in the treatment of mice challenged intranasally with vesicular stomatitis virus (VSV). Proc. Soc. exp. Biol. Med. *138:* 301–307 (1971).

16 De Somer, P.; Edy, V. G.; Billiau, A.: Interferon-induced skin reactivity in man. Lancet *ii:* 47–48 (1977).

17 Desmyter, J.; Ray, M. B.; De Groote, J.; Bradburne, A. F.; Desmet, V. J.; Edy, V. G.; Billiau, A.; De Somer, P.; Mortelmans, J.: Administration of human fibroblast interferon in chronic hepatitis-B infection. Lancet *ii:* 645–647 (1976).

18 Edy, V.G.; Billiau, A.; De Somer, P.: Non-appearance of injected fibroblast interferon in the circulation. Lancet *ii:* 451–452 (1978).

19 Gresser, I.; Fontaine-Brouty-Boye, D.; Bouraly, C.; Thomas, M. T.: A comparison of the efficacy of endogenous, exogenous, and combined endogenous-exogenous interferon in the treatment of mice infected with encephalomyocarditis virus. Proc. Soc. exp. Biol. Med. *130:* 236–242 (1969).

20 Gresser, I.; Bouraly-Maury, C.: Inhibition by interferon preparations of a solid

malignant tumor and pulmonary metastases in mice. Nature new Biol. *236:* 78–79 (1972).

21 Gresser, I.; Tovey, M. G.; Bouraly-Maury, C.: Efficacy of exogenous interferon treatment initiated after onset of multiplication of vesicular stomatitis virus in the brains of mice. J. gen. Virol. *27:*395–398 (1975).

22 Gresser, I.; Tovey, M. G.: Antitumor effects of interferon. Biochim. biophys. Acta *516:*231–247 (1978).

23 Heine, J. W.; De Ley, M.; Van Damme, J.; Billiau, A.; De Somer, P.: Human fibroblast interferon purified to homogeneity by a two-step procedure. Ann. N. Y. Acad. Sci. *350:*364–373 (1980).

24 Heine, J. W.; Van Damme, J.; De Ley, M.; Billiau, A.; De Somer, P.: Purification of human fibroblast interferon by zinc-chelate chromatography. J. gen. Virol. (in press, 1981).

25 Heremans, H.; Billiau, A.; De Somer, P.: Interferon in experimental viral infections in mice: Tissue levels resulting from the virus infection and from exogenous therapy. Infect. Immunity *30:*513–522 (1980).

26 Hitchcock, G.; Porterfield, J. S.: The production of interferon in brains of mice infected with arthropod-bone virus. Virology *13:*363–365 (1961).

27 Horoszewicz, J. S.; Leong, S. S.; Ito, M.; Buffett, R. F.; Karakousis, C.; Holyoke, E.; Job, L.; Dölen, J. G.; Carter, W. A.: Human fibroblast interferon in human neoplasia: Clinical and laboratory study. Cancer Treatm. Rep. *62:* 1899–1906 (1978).

28 Horoszewicz, J. S.; Leong, S. S.; Dolen, J. G.; Holyoke, E. D.; Karakousis, C.; Nemoto, T.; Wajsman, L. Z.; Freeman, A. I.; Aungst, C.W.; Henderson, E.; Carter, W. A.: Purified human fibroblast interferon and neoplasia: Pharmacokinetic studies and selective antiproliferative properties *in vivo*. In: Amanullah, Hill, Dorn, Interferon: Properties and Clinical Uses, pp. 661–666 (Leland Fikes Foundation Press of the Wadley Institutes, Dallas 1980).

29 Kassel, R. L.: Carcinolytic effects of interferon. Clin. Obstet. Gynec. *13:*910–927 (1970).

30 Lucero, M. A.; Fridman, W. H.; Provost, M. A.; Billardon, C.; Pouillart, P.; Dumont, J.; Falcoff, E.: Effect of various interferons on the spontaneous cytotoxicity exerted by lymphocytes from normal and tumor-bearing patients. Cancer Res. *41:*294–299 (1981).

31 McPherson, T. A.; Tan, Y. H.: Phase-I pharmacotoxicology study of human fibroblast interferon in human cancers. J. natn. Cancer Inst. *65:*75–79 (1980).

32 Nagata, S.; Mantei, N.; Weissman, C.: The structure of one of the eight or more distinct chromosomal genes for human interferon-α. Nature *287:*401–408 (1980).

33 Proceedings Conference on Clinical Potentials of Interferons in Viral Diseases and Malignant Tumors, Oiso, Japan, December 1980 (Japan Medical Research Foundation, in press, 1981).

34 Schouten, T. J.; Bos, J. H.: Interferon, juveniele larynx papillomen en de wenselijkheid van een Nederlandse productie van interferon. Ned. Tijdschr. Geneesk. *124:*1650–1651 (1980).

35 Sehgal, P. B.; Sagar, A. D.: Heterogeneity of poly(I):poly(C)-induced human fibroblast interferon mRNA species. Nature *288:*95–98 (1980).

36 Treuner, J.; Niethammer, D.; Dannecker, G.; Hagmann, R.; Neef, V.; Hofschneider, P. H.: Successful treatment of nasopharyngeal carcinoma with interferon. Lancet *i:*817–818 (1980).

37 Van Damme, J.; De Ley, M.; Claeys, J.; Billiau, A.; Vermylen, C.; De Somer, P.: Interferon induced in human leukocytes by concanavalin-A: Isolation and characterization of γ- and β-type components. Eur. J. Immunol. (submitted 1981).

38 Vilček, J.: Production of interferon by newborn and adult mice infected with Sindbis virus. Virology *22:*651–652 (1964).
39 Weimar, W.; Schellekens, H.; Lameijer, L. D. F.; Masurel, N.; Edy, V. G.; Billiau, A.; De Somer, P.: Double-blind study of interferon administration in renal transplant recipients. Eur. J. clin. Invest. *8:*255–258 (1978).
40 Weimar, W.; Heijtink, R. A.; Schalm, S. W.; Schellekens, H.: Differential effects of fibroblast and leukocyte interferon in HBsAg-positive chronic active hepatitis. Eur. J. clin. Invest. *9:*151–154 (1979).

P. de Somer, MD, Rega Institute – K. U. Leuven, Minderbroedersstraat 10, B-3000 Leuven

Corneal Interferon Treatment of Herpetic Keratitis in Monkeys

D. Neumann-Haefelin[1], *R. Sundmacher*[2], *K. Cantell*[3]

[1] Institut für Virologie, Zentrum für Hygiene, Universität Freiburg, FRG
[2] Universitäts-Augenklinik, Freiburg, FRG
[3] Central Public Health Laboratory, Helsinki, Finland

This short review of our work on experimental keratitis in monkeys may be useful, in part, as an introduction to the clinical interferon studies in ophthalmology, presented in the following paper of this volume (*Sundmacher,* The Clinical Value of Interferon in Ocular Viral Diseases).

Most primate studies, human and non-human, concerned with the antiviral effect of interferon have faced two main difficulties: firstly, interferon rarely confers any benefit once the symptoms of viral infection have developed; secondly, whenever beneficial effects are suspected, their assessment and control is difficult. This is different with herpetic keratitis, at least with the epithelial form.

The advantages of antiviral studies in corneal disease are: easy assessment of symptoms, feasibility of virus isolation from the corneal surface for control of virus-specificity, and the convenience of applying the antiviral agent, as the corneal epithelium is readily accessible for topical treatment. The conjunctival space allows rather well-defined, reproducible, and economic dosage of interferon simply with eye drops.

Another important argument for interferon studies in herpetic keratitis is the fact that, in man, the disease is generally caused by recurrent herpes simplex virus infection. The present hypothesis of herpetic recurrency is well in accordance with abundant experimental and clinical evidence [1, 6]. From clinical observations we also conclude that release of virus from the nerve cell is not restricted to a short period before onset of epithelial disease, but that prolonged neurogenic virus production is one of the factors determining the course of dendritic keratitis. Permanent or repeated virus shedding from the nerve endings is suspected to delay spontaneous epithelial healing, or to induce early relapses. This situation could offer an excellent chance for interferon "therapy", which would then be nothing else than protection of still uninfected epithelial tissue from continued neurogenic infection.

Experimental herpes simplex virus (HSV) inoculation into the monkey cornea causes only nonrecurrent primary infection. However, the value of antiviral measures in the animal can be regarded as predictive for clinical evaluations. In addition to the technical advantages, this has made viral keratitis a favored model for in vivo studies of antiviral interferon activity. Early experiments in rabbits and man, by the groups of *Cantell* [2], *Jones* [4], and *Finter* [3] in the 1960s, rendered controversial results. Nevertheless, experiments in monkeys were resumed by *Kaufman et al.* [5, 10] some years later. These studies clearly showed the protective effect of prophylactically administered human interferon against experimental herpes simplex virus infection of the cornea.

Our own task – with clinical studies in mind – was to confirm and to quantify this effect in monkeys.

We first attempted to overcome the limitation of small numbers, which is a critical point in all experimental primate studies. Therefore, we performed interferon treatment (daily evaluations by virus isolation and slitlamp microscopy) in the right eye, and mock-interferon treatment in the left eye of each monkey (cercopithecus aetiops), both eyes being identically infected. (The infectivity of herpes simplex virus type 1 inocula ranged from 10^6 to 2×10^7 $TCID_{50}$ per 0.1 ml). Thus the efficacy of herpes-virus infection can be controlled individually in each animal. Initial pilot studies indicated, and this has been verified in further experiments, that the eyes of one animal react independently as far as viral infection and interferon treatment are concerned [7].

Table I reviews the results of a comparative study [8] of human leukocyte interferon (IFN-α) and fibroblast interferon (IFN-β). In both parts of the experiment, all control eyes developed keratitis and rendered positive herpes-virus isolations. Acceptably active interferon, regardless of its origin, protected all of the treated eyes from infection and disease. With activity one magnitude lower, the protective effect was only partial. Further reduction made the benefit of inter-

Table I. Infection by human IFN-α and IFN-β from HSV-1 infection and keratitis in African green monkeys (cercopithecus aetiops)

IFN-activity (ref. u./ml)	IFN-α-treated eyes*		IFN-β-treated eyes*	
	Keratitis	HSV recovered	Keratitis	HSV recovered
1.9×10^6	0/4**	0/4	0/4	0/4
1.9×10^5	1/4	1/4	2/4	2/4
1.9×10^4	3/4	3/4	4/4	3/4
1.9×10^3	4/4	4/4	4/4	3/3
Mock-IFN	16/16	16/16	16/16	16/16

* 0.05 ml, 13 h before, 0, and 24 h post infection
** No. of eyes positive per number of eyes studied in the respective group

feron rather marginal, and in the last group, where only 190 reference units of interferon were given per 0.1 ml in a single dose, no difference to the controls could be ovserved.

Beside clear data defining the requirements for reliable corneal protection, this experiment provided the information that interferon-α and interferon-β of equal in vitro titer (determined in diploid human fibroblast cultures, challenged with vesicular stomatitis virus) may also be equally effective in vivo. To our knowledge, this has not been demonstrated in any other primate study so far.

Of course, this conclusion is only admissible for topical interferon application, whereas in the case of systemic treatment, the situation may be completely changed due to different molecular properties and different pharmacokinetics [9].

We used this model in some additional experiments (table II), and could show that leukocyte interferon still works under poorer conditions, as for instance on the steroid-prechallenged cornea [12], or without handicapping of herpes virus, i.e. starting interferon treatment simultaneously with infection, and not before [7]. In the same experiment, we tried to go one step further, giving the initial dose of interferon 6 h post infection. At this point, we were unsuccessful. Once established, the herpes-virus infection proceeded and resulted in keratitis and virus shedding. Due to the benign and self-limiting nature of the disease in monkeys, curative effects of the post-infectional interferon schedule could not be assessed. However, the lack of direct therapeutic potency of interferon was not unexpected

Table II. Different schedules of IFN-α treatment for prevention of HSV-1-induced keratitis in African green monkeys

Begin of treatment	IFN-activity (ref. u./ single dose)	Keratitis	HSV recovered
Preinfectional*	1×10^4	1/4	1/4
	1×10^5	0/4	0/4
	Mock-IFN	8/8	8/8
Preinfectional** and steroids***	1.4×10^5	0/6	0/6
	Mock-IFN	6/6	6/6
Simultaneous**** with infection	2×10^4	0/2	0/2
Postinfectional*****	2×10^4	4/4	4/4
	Mock-IFN	6/6	6/6

* 13 h before, 0, and 24 h post infection, 0.05 ml IFN
** 15 h before, 0, 24, 48, and 72 h post infection, 0.05 ml IFN
*** 2 days before to 3 days post infection dexamethason-phosphate 2 × daily
**** 0, 12, 24, 36, 48, 60, 72, and 90 h post infection, 0.150 ml IFN
***** 6, 18, 32, 48, 60, 72, 84, 96 h post infection, 0.150 ml IFN

and is quite in line with our experiences in human dendritic keratitis [11, 13].

There are other problem areas in human ophthalmology where a beneficial effect of interferon would be desirable, and this encouraged further studies in monkeys. We refer to the problems of herpes-virus activity *beneath* the intact epithelium, which results in the initiation of dendritic recurrences, and is suspected to be one of the causal factors of deep or stromal keratitis. As neither endogenous herpetic recurrences nor stromal complications of simple exogenous infection occur in monkeys, we modified our model by injecting herpes-virus into the monkey cornea. This type of infection results in a rather violent stromal keratitis, in most cases accompanied by iritis.

The data of table III show that we could not prevent stromal disease by different modes of interferon treatment. Neither eye drops, applied in some animals after partial removal of the epithelial barrier, nor intracorneally injected interferon effected any significant modulation of stromal infection when compared with mock treatment.

Table III. Different modes of corneal IFN-α treatment of African green monkeys infected intracorneally by injection of 10^7 $TCID_{50}$ HSV 1 in 0.03 ml

Mode of treatment*	IFN-activity (ref. u./ single dose)	Occurrence of stromal HSV infection
Eye drops onto intact corneal epithelium	3×10^5	4 / 4
	Mock-IFN	4 / 4
Eye drops after epithelial abrasio	3×10^5	3 / 3
	Mock-IFN	3 / 3
Intracorneal injection	3×10^5	4 / 4
	Mock-IFN	4 / 4

* 13 h before, 0, 24, 48, and 72 h post infection

Some differences were observed, however, as far as side effects of interferon treatment are concerned. While the minimal side effects of epithelial treatment were negligible, absence of the epithelial barrier and intracorneal or even subconjunctival injection of interferon seemed to add non-viral (toxic?) problems to the infected eyes of some animals. The partially purified interferon that we used for our experiments is probably not suitable for this type of evaluation. Future studies will show whether preparations of highly purified interferon will be more easily tolerated.

In fact, well-tolerated interferon treatment of stromal processes may have some beneficial effect *beside* the antiviral activity. The immune-modulatory function of interferon could be useful by modifying the non-viral pathogenic events that are thought to play an important role in human stromal keratitis of herpetic origin.

References

1 Baringer, J. R.; Swoveland, P.: Recovery of herpes simplex virus from human tigeminal ganglions. New Eng. J. Med. *288:* 648 – 650 (1973).

2 Cantell, K.; Tommila, V.: Effect of interferon on experimental vaccina and herpes simplex virus infections in rabbits' eyes. Lancet *ii:* 628 – 684 (1960).

3 Finter, N. B.: Exogenous interferon in animals and its clinical implications. Archs. intern. Med. *126:* 147 – 157 (1970).

4 Jones, B. R.; Galbraith, J. E. K.; Al-Hussaini, M. K.: Vaccinal keratitis treated with interferon. Lancet *i:* 875 – 879 (1962).
5 Kaufman, H. E.; Ellison, E. D.; Centifanto, Y. M.: Difference in interferon response and protection from ocular virus infection in rabbits and monkeys. Am. J. Ophthal. *74:* 89 – 92 (1972).
6 Klein, R. J.: Pathogenic mechanisms of recurrent herpes simplex virus infections. Archs Virol. *51:* 1 – 13 (1976).
7 Neumann-Haefelin, D.; Sundmacher, R.; Sauter, B.; Karges, H. E.; Manthey, K. F.: Effect of human leukocyte interferon on vaccina- and herpes-virus-infected cell cultures and monkey corneas. Infect. Immunity *12:* 148 – 155 (1975).
8 Neumann-Haefelin, D.; Sundmacher, R.; Skoda, R.; Cantell, K.: Comparative evaluation of human leukocyte and fibroblast interferon in the prevention of herpes simplex virus keratitis in a monkey model. Infect. Immunity *17:* 468 – 470 (1977).
9 Stewart, W. E., II: The interferon system (Springer-Verlag, Wien 1979).
10 Sugar, J.; Kaufman, H. E.; Varnell, E. D.: Effect of exogenous interferon on herpetic keratitis in rabbits and monkeys. Investigative Ophth. *12:* 378 – 380 (1973).
11 Sundmacher, R.; Neumann-Haefelin, D.; Cantell, K.: Successful treatment of dendritic keratitis with human leukocyte interferon. A controlled clinical study. Graefes Arch. klin. exp. Ophthal. *201:* 39 – 45 (1976).
12 Sundmacher, R.; Cantell, K.; Haug, P.; Neumann-Haefelin, D.: Inteferon-Prophylaxe von Dendritica-Rezidiven bei lokaler Steroidtherapie. Ber. Versamm. dt. ophthal. Ges. *75:* 344 – 346 (1977).
13 Sundmacher, R.; Cantell, K.; Haug, P.; Neumann-Haefelin, D.: Role of debridement and interferon in the treatment of dendritic keratitis. Graefes Arch. klin. exp. Ophthal. *207:* 77 – 82 (1978).

Dr. D. Neumann-Haefelin, Institut für Virologie im Zentrum für Hygiene der Universität Freiburg, Hermann-Herder-Str. 11, D-7800 Freiburg

The Clinical Value of Interferon in Ocular Viral Diseases

R. Sundmacher[1], *D. Neumann-Haefelin*[1], *K. Cantell*[2]

[1] Augenklinik und Institut für Virologie, Universität Freiburg, FRG
[2] Central Public Health Laboratory, Helsinki, Finland

Viral diseases of the anterior segment of the eye offer unique advantages for the study of antiviral agents. First, the close observation of the viral lesions with the slitlamp (biomicroscope) allows the discrimination of even slight morphological changes, and thus the control of the clinical course of the disease is precise and reliable. Secondly, viral cultures may be easily obtained – at least from surface lesions – and may serve as a valuable control for clinical judgment. Thirdly, viral diseases of surface lesions of the conjunctiva and cornea can be treated by topical therapy without the limitations of systemic applications. Deep lesions, however, especially if they are covered by an intact corneal epithelium, do not generally lend themselves to topical treatment, and some of them do not respond to eye drops because of pharmacokinetic problems.

The major threat to vision after birth comes from herpes viruses (herpes simplex virus, varicella zoster virus, cytomegalovirus), and adenoviruses which lead periodically to epidemics with disabling diseases. Only part of this broad spectrum of diseases has as yet been adequately studied in respect of interferon treatment; and only herpes simplex virus disease of the corneal epithelium (dendritic keratitis) has been a successful target (for reviews see [2, 14]). As yet we have not been able to confirm positive reports on interferon therapy of epidemic keratoconjunctivitis which is caused by adenoviruses [5]. A trial with systemic interferon therapy in a child with severe connatal cytomegalovirus eye infection failed [16]. With interferon treatment of intraocular zoster infections, the results appear more promising. The pathophysiology of this disease, however, is complicated and, up to now, the clinical value of systemic interferon therapy in ophthalmic zoster cannot be regarded as established [15]. These negative results may appear disappointing. One has to consider, however, that in the case of dendritic keratitis we also had negative results in the beginning [9] and have nonetheless obtained clinically significant results which we would like to discuss in some detail.

For treatment of dendritic keratitis, two forms of therapy exist which are both quite active; first, debridement of the diseased epithelium; and, secondly, topical therapy with synthetic antiviral agents. For interferon to be of clinical interest, it should at least meet, or better surpass, the therapeutic efficiency of these two forms of therapy. This is clearly not the case. The therapeutic activity of interferon, when used as the sole therapeutic agent, is quite poor – if it exists at all [9, 11]; and the results of other authors confirm that it is not advisable to use interferon monotherapy for dendritic keratitis [2, 6, 18].

In combination, however, with an antiviral therapy, which in itself is very potent, interferon brings about a further significant improvement of therapeutic results. This was first established for the combination of interferon with debridement [1, 7, 8] and thereafter for the combination of interferon with the topical antiherpetic agent trifluorothymidine (TFT) [12, 14]. The combination of TFT with human leukocyte interferon (HLI) at 30×10^6 U/ml resulted in such a tremendous improvement of therapy that, at present, it seems unlikely that any further substantial progress can be achieved [14]. The only disadvantage would be the need for a very potent interferon preparation. We, therefore, performed a new study in an attempt to reduce the amount of interferon needed without losing clinical activity.

Patients and Methods

Clinical diagnosis, randomization, and viral controls were as described previously [14]. The patients received either one drop of HLI_{IA} and 10 min later a second drop of HLI_{IB} or HLI_{IIA} and HLI_{IIB}, respectively. From the day of fluorescein-negative healing, the treatment was changed to 2 drops of either HLI_{IB} or HLI_{IIB}, respectively, for a further 3 days and then stopped. Five drops of TFT 1% were administered daily from the beginning and continued for 3 days after cessation of interferon treatment and then also stopped. Artificial tears were added when a dry-eye syndrome complicated the disease. The code was as follows:

HLI_{IA} = human leukocyte interferon (10×10^6 U/ml)
HLI_{IB} = placebo (human serum albumin)
HLI_{IIA} = human leukocyte interferon (30×10^6 U/ml)
HLI_{IIB} = human leukocyte interferon (30×10^6 U/ml)

In summary one patient group was treated with only 1 drop daily of HLI (10×10^6 U/ml) up to the day of fluorescein-negative healing of the corneal epithelium. The second group received 2 drops daily of the more potent preparation (30×10^6 U/ml), and this regime was continued for 3 days longer than the first group.

Results

Only those patients were accepted for final evaluation who had delivered at least one positive viral culture. This was done in order to be quite sure of the viral nature of the disease treated, because non-viral (metaherpetic) diseases may mimic viral diseases. There were 24 patients with proven viral diseases who were treated with HLI (10×10^6 U/ml), and 27 patients who received HLI (30×10^6 U/ml). Up to day 3 of the combination treatment, there was absolutely no difference between the healing curves of both groups (fig. 1). Thereafter, a clinical difference was noted which did not quite reach the level of statistical significance. The virus-shedding curves (fig. 2) exhibited no difference whatsoever. The amount of interferon used is shown in table I.

Discussion

Prior investigation showed that a combination therapy of dendritic keratitis with TFT plus highly potent HLI (30×10^6 U/ml) improved therapeutic results considerably whereas a low potent interferon (1×10^6 U/ml) improved the results only slightly and failed to reach statistical significance [14]. Our new study shows that the amount of interferon can be reduced 9-fold without losing much clinical activity. We applied 1 drop of HLI (10×10^6 U/ml) for an average

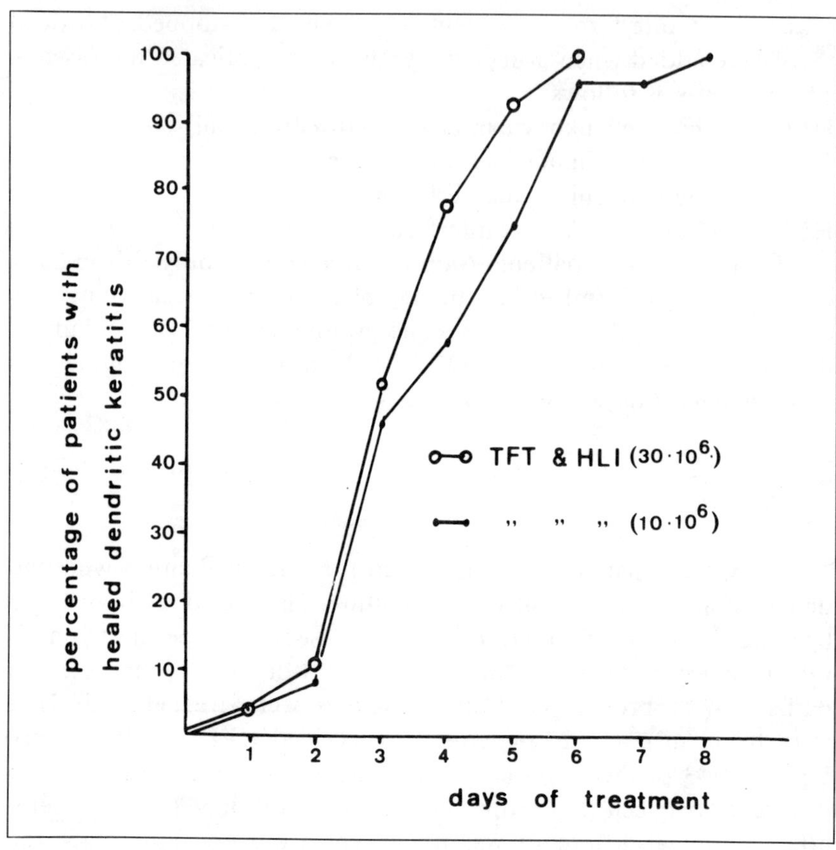

Figure 1. Healing of the corneal epithelium in dendritic keratitis.

of 4.2 days, and 2 drops of HLI (30×10^6 U/ml) for an average of 6.6 days (table I). It seems reasonable to advocate, therefore, the regime with the lower potent HLI (10×10^6 U/ml) as long as the production of the more potent one is difficult.

On the other hand, it still seems preferable to use the more potent HLI. It is true that in this study no statistically significant difference was found; on the other hand, however, if one analyzes our accumulated data on therapy of dendritic keratitis with TFT-HLI combinations, one finds a clear dose-response relationship between HLI titers and clinical activity; and this is also true for the difference between 10×10^6 U/ml and 30×10^6 U/ml [17].

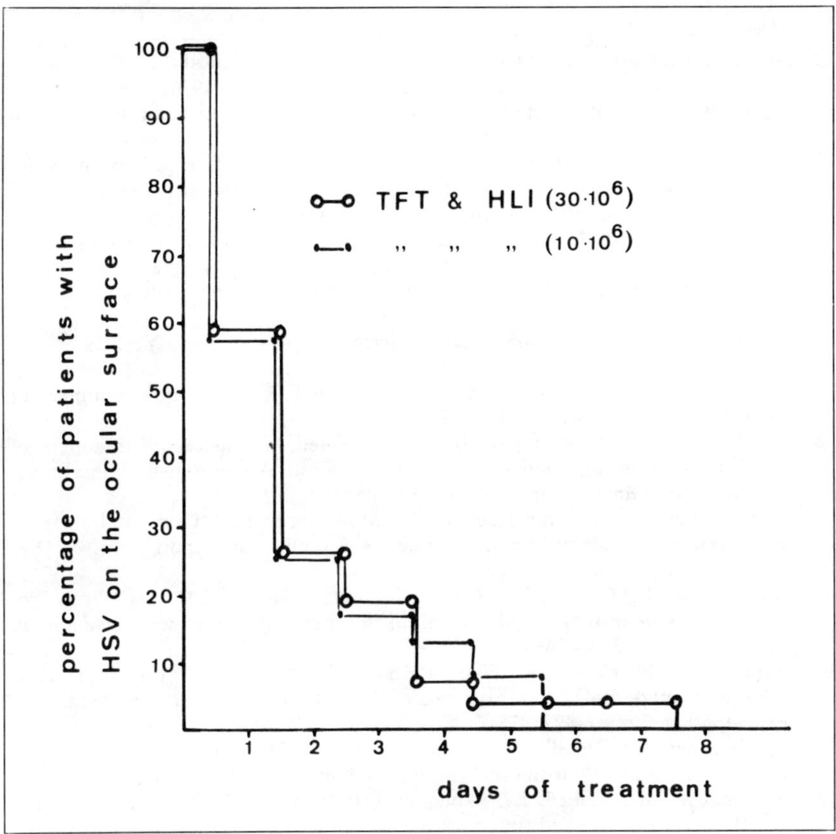

Figure 2. Virus isolations from the cul-de sac in dendritic keratitis.

Table 1. Quantity of interferon employed

	Human leukocyte interferon (U/ml)	
	10×10^6	30×10^6
Drops (0.05 ml) per day	1	2
Healing time (days)	4.2	3.3
Time of HLI application (days)	4.2	6.3
HLI (ml) used per patient	0.21	0.63
HLI (U) used per patient	2.1×10^6	18.9×10^6

References

1 Jones, B. R.; Coster, D. J.; Falcon, M. G.; Cantell, K.: Topical therapy of ulcerative herpetic keratitis with human interferon. Lancet *ii:* 128 (1976).

2 Jones, B. R.: Human interferon in topical therapy of herpetic keratitis. In: Sundmacher, Herpetic eye diseases, pp. 395 – 400 (J. F. Bergmann, München 1981).

3 Kaufman, H. E.; Meyer, R. F.; Laibson, P. R.; Waltman, S. R.; Nesburn, A. B.; Shuster, J. J.: Human leukocyte interferon for the prevention of recurrences of herpetic keratitis. J. Infect. Dis., suppl. 133, pp. A165 – A168 (1976).

4 Neumann-Haefelin, D.; Sundmacher, R.; Skoda, R.; Cantell, K.: Comparative evaluation of human leukocyte and fibroblast interferon in the prevention of herpes simplex virus keratitis in a monkey model. Infect. Immunity *17:* 468 – 470 (1977).

5 Revel, M.: Discussion remark. Second interferon workshop, New York 1979.

6 Shiota, H.: Discussion remark to Jones, B. R. (see [2]).

7 Sundmacher, R.; Neumann-Haefelin, D.; Cantell, K.: Interferon treatment of dendritic keratitis. Lancet *i:* 1406 (1976).

8 Sundmacher, R.; Neumann-Haefelin, D.; Cantell, K.: Successful treatment of dendritic keratitis with human leukocyte interferon. A controlled clinical study. Graefes Arch. klin. exp. Ophthal. *201:* 39 – 45 (1976).

9 Sundmacher, R.; Neumann-Haefelin, D.; Manthey, K. F.; Müller, O.: Interferon in treatment of dendritic keratitis in humans. A preliminary report. J. Infect. Dis., suppl. 133, pp. A160 – A164 (1976).

10 Sundmacher, R.; Cantell, K.; Haug, P.; Neumann-Haefelin, D.: Interferon-Prophylaxe von Dendritica-Rezidiven bei lokaler Steroidtherapie. Ber. Versamm. dt. ophthal. Ges. *75:* 344 – 346 (1977).

11 Sundmacher, R.; Cantell, K.; Haug, P.; Neumann-Haefelin, D.: Role of debridement and interferon in the treatment of dendritic keratitis. Graefes Arch. klin. exp. Ophthal. *207:* 77–82 (1978).

12 Sundmacher, R.; Cantell, K.; Neumann-Haefelin, D.: Combination therapy of dendritic keratitis with trifluorothymidine and interferon. Lancet *ii:* 687 (1978).

13 Sundmacher, R.; Cantell, K.; Skoda, R.; Hallermann, C.; Neumann-Haefelin, D.: Human leukocyte and fibroblast interferon in a combination therapy of dendritic keratitis. Graefes Arch. klin. exp. Ophthal. *208:* 229 – 233 (1978).

14 Sundmacher, R.; Neumann-Haefelin, D.; Cantell, K.: Therapy and prophylaxis of dendritic keratitis with topical human interferon. In: Sundmacher, Herpetic eye diseases, pp. 401 – 407 (J. F. Bergmann, München 1981).

15 Sundmacher, R.; Neumann-Haefelin, D.; Cantell, K.: Trials with interferon in ophthalmic zoster. In: Sundmacher, Herpetic eye diseases, pp. 465 – 468 (J. F. Bergmann, München 1981).

16 Sundmacher, R.; Neumann-Haefelin, D.; Mattes, A.; Cantell, K.: Connatal monosymptomatic corneal endothelitis by cytomegalovirus. In: Sundmacher, Herpetic eye diseases, pp. 501 – 504 (J. F. Bergmann, München 1981).

17 Sundmacher, R.; Cantell, K.; Neumann-Haefelin, D.: Evaluation of interferon in ocular viral diseases. In: De Maeyer, Galasso, Schellekens, The Biology of the Interferon System, (pp. 343 – 350 Elsevier/North-Holland Biomedical Press, Amsterdam 1981).

18 Uchida, Y.; Kaneko, M.; Yamanishi, R.; Kobayashi, S.: Effect of human fibroblast interferon on dendritic keratitis. In: Sundmacher, Herpetic eye diseases, pp. 409 – 413 (J. F. Bergmann, München 1981).

Doz. Dr. Rainer Sundmacher, Klinikum der Albert-Ludwigs-Universität, Univ.-Augenklinik, Killianstr. 5, D-7800 Freiburg

Human Interferon-Beta in Chronic Active Hepatitis B: Preliminary Data of a Controlled Trial*

R. Müller[1], *F. Deinhardt*[2], *G. Frösner*[2], *H. P. Hofschneider*[3], *H. Klein*[1], *F. W. Schmidt*[1], *W. Siegert*[4], *E. Wille*[1], *I. Vido*[1]

[1] Abt. f. Gastroenterologie und Hepatologie, Zentrum Innere Medizin, Medizinische Hochschule Hannover, FRG
[2] Max von Pettenkofer-Institut, München, FRG
[3] Max Planck-Institut für Biochemie, Martinsried bei München, FRG
[4] 3. Medizinische Klinik der Ludwig Maximilians Universität, München, FRG

Introduction

Impaired interferon production has been suggested to be responsible for the failure of patients with hepatitis B antigen (HBsAg) positive chronic active liver disease (CALD) to overcome persistent hepatitis B virus (HBV) infection [5, 8, 14, 15, 19]. This hypothesis had led to several trials on interferon therapy in chronic active hepatitis B (CAHB), a disease, which, in general, continuously progresses to liver cirrhosis and may end up in hepatoma. The interferons which have been applied were human leukocyte interferon (HuIFN-α) and human fibroblast interferon (HuIFN-β) [1, 2, 3, 4, 7, 10, 16, 17, 18]. The most comprehensive data available on HuIFN-α, used as single-agent treatment regimen, have been reported by *Merigan et al.* on 16 individuals [11, 12]. Patients completing treatment revealed 3 different types of responses:

- A permanent reduction of Dane particles, HBe- und HBs- antigens to below the level of detection even on cessation of therapy was observed in 2 females (response type 1).
- A permanent reduction of Dane particles and HBeAg, a partial reduction of HBsAg, and a disappearance of HBcAg from the liver tissue were seen in another 3 patients (response type 2).

* Supported by the Ministry of Research and Technology, Bonn, FRG

- A partial reduction of Dane particles during treatment only and no change in HBsAg was reported in 12 patients (response type 3).

Similar findings were established by others in an even smaller number of patients who have undergone HuIFN-α treatment [18].

Data obtained with treatment of HuIFN-β in patients with CAHB have been variable. Some investigators have reported a partial suppression of HBV-infection, while others failed to confirm any consistent effect on the indices of HBV-replication in CAHB [1, 2, 10, 17]. This difference to HuIFN-α was suspected to be most likely due to the fact that effective levels of HuIFN-β did not reach the liver, since no measurable interferon blood levels could be detected on intramuscular or subcutaneous injection of HuIFN-β in contrast to HuIFN-α.

Material and Methods

In 1978 a multicenter controlled trial was set up to evaluate the effect that long-term dosage of HuIFN-β exerts on intravenous administration in patients with CAHB. This trial is not yet completed. Preliminary data presented here include observations in 1 female and 10 male patients having been treated with HuIFN-β kindly provided by Dr. Rentschler GmbH (Laupheim, West Germany).

Patients selected for trial had to fulfill the following criteria:

- chronic active hepatitis B with persistently abnormal liver-function tests for at least 1 year;
- demonstration of chronic aggressive hepatitis on biopsy;
- presence of HBsAg and HBeAg in serum; and
- no immunosuppressive therapy during the observation period.

The observation period covered 15 months: 6 months prior to treatment, 6 months of HuIFN-β administration, and 3 months of post-treatment observations. In the first 5 patients HuIFN-β was administered intravenously according to the following schedule:

- 10 Mio. U per day for 3 days;
- 6 Mio. U per day another 3 days;
- 4 Mio. U per day for 3 weeks; and
- 4 Mio. U every 3 days for 5 months.

In 2 patients out of this group, HuIFN-β dosage was discontinued after a 4-week period of treatment, because of jaundice and encephalopathia in one individual and increasing fatigue in the other. Both patients were excluded from the study. In the remaining 6 patients treatment regimen was modified. Intravenous doses of 10 Mio. U per day were given for 1 month and subsequently 10 Mio. U every 3 days for 5 months.

Liver-function tests and HBV-markers, including DNAP-activity, HBsAg and HBeAg in the serum, were measured once a month for 6 months prior to treatment, every two weeks during HuIFN-β dosage, and once a month during post-treatment observations. The same serological testing was done in the controls once a month for 15 months. Liver biopsies were performed in patients undergoing HuIFN-β treatment for demonstration of HBcAg, HBsAg, and delta-Ag. Biopsies were done before, 4 weeks after, and 6 months after onset of HuIFN-β treatment. No liver biopsies were performed in the controls.

DNAP-activity was measured by incorporation of 3 HTTP into cores of partially purified Dane particles as described by *Kaplan et al.* [9]. HBeAg titers were measured by EIA and RIA (HBe™, Abbott Lab. Chicago, Ill.), and HBsAg determinations were performed by RIA (Ausria II, Abbott Lab. Chicago, Ill.) and quantitatively by a modification of Laurell immunoelectrophoresis [6]. HBcAg, HBsAb, and delta-Ag were demonstrated in unfixed, air-dried cryostat sections of liver biopsies by a highly purified human FITC-labeled anti-HBc-IgG, anti-HBs-immunoglobulin, and anti-delta-immunoglobulin, respectively. The FITC-labeled anti-delta-immunoglobulin was kindly provided by Dr. M. Rizzetto (Turino, Italy).

Interferon blood levels were measured by a micro-CPE reduction assay with the Indiana strain of VSV.

Results

6 individuals had fulfilled the trials procedures by 1 March 1981. The last 3 patients are undergoing post-treatment observations. Circulating interferon blood levels could be detected in patients treated and were found to be as high as 360 U/ml 5 min after injection of 10 Mio U of HuIFN-β. The response to HuIFN-β is summarized in figure 1. A significant, but transient, decline of HBV-specific DNAP-

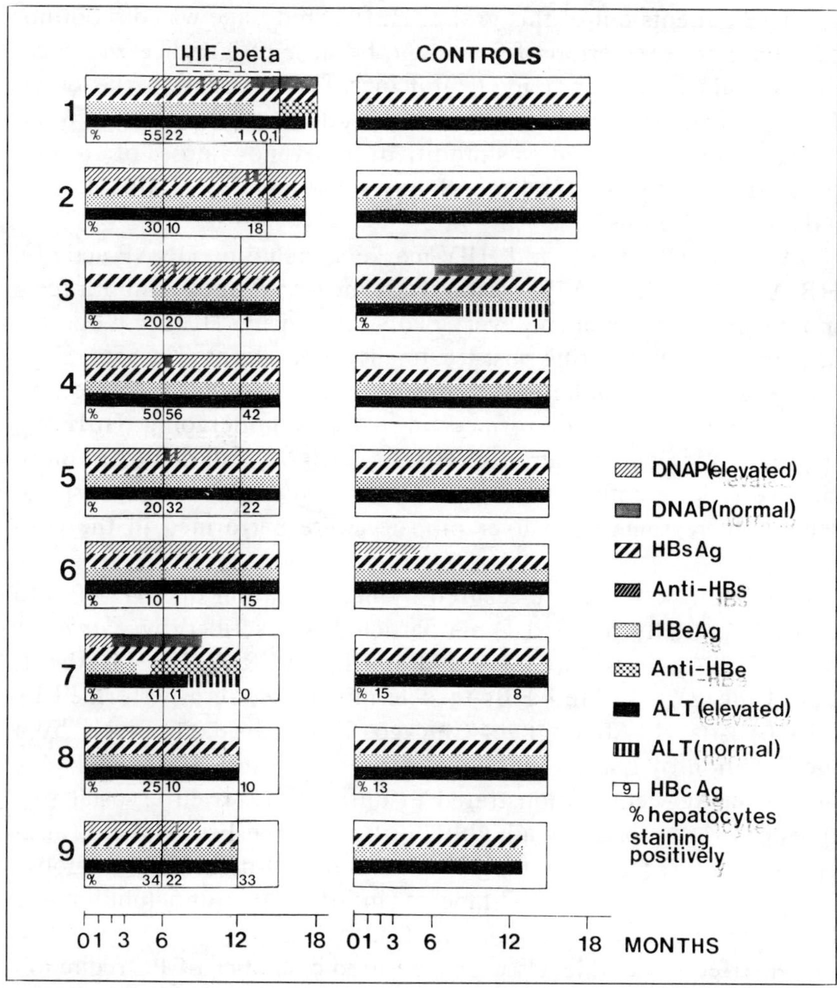

Fig. 1. HBV-markers and ALT-activity in 9 patients and 9 controls: Response to i. v. administration of HuIFN-β. Presence of the various markers is indicated by different symbols. Missing symbols of DNAP-activity in controls and treated patients indicate that sera are still undergoing investigation.

activity was observed in all patients having undergone HuIFN-β therapy. In 6 individuals DNAP-activity temporarily decreased to below the level of detection. The main drop occurred during the first 4 weeks of treatment when HuIFN-β was injected at daily intervals (fig. 2).

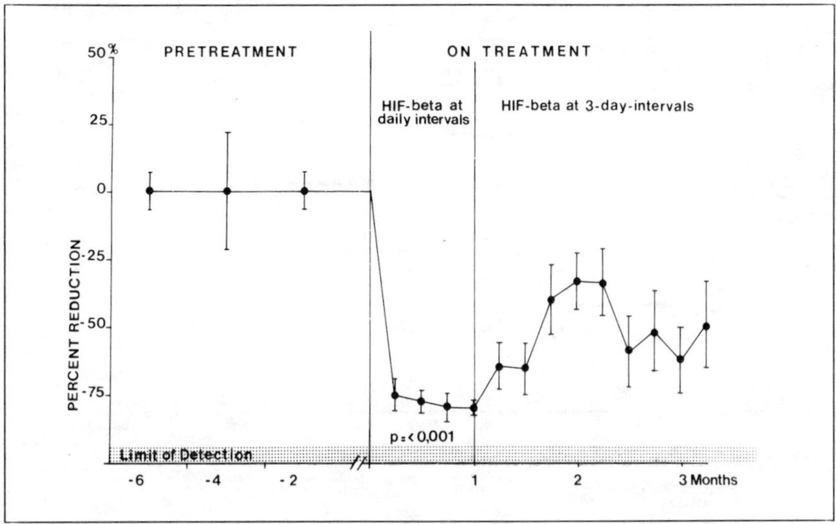

Fig. 2. Percent reduction of DNAP-activity after onset of HuIFN-β treatment. Mean values of DNAP-activity of each patient's pretreatment series of sera are regarded as 100%. Mean-values (●) of percent reduction and standard error of the mean (SEM) are depicted for the first 13 weeks of HuIFN-β treatment.

The most remarkable changes on the expression of HBV-markers in chronic HBV-infection were observed in patient 1 and patient 7.

DNAP-activity in patient 1 decreased to below the level of detection 6 months after onset of HuIFN-β treatment. 2 weeks later HBeAg disappeared from the serum and, after an interval of additional two months, the patient had developed anti-HBe. For the first time in 8 years of consistent abnormal liver-function tests, enzyme activities of this patient declined to normal values during the last month of post-treatment observation (fig. 3).

Essentially the same changes were seen in patient 7 except that they occurred prior to HuIFN-β treatment. This incomplete suppression of HBV-infection was not completely recognized during pretreatment observation when the patient was selected for trial. In retrospect it is considered a response to rapid withdrawal of immunosuppressive therapy which the patient had undergone before entering the study. An one-step withdrawal of immunosuppressive drugs in CAHB may release exaggerated host-recovery responses, which exert a suppressive effect on chronic HBV-infection [13]. Therefore the dis-

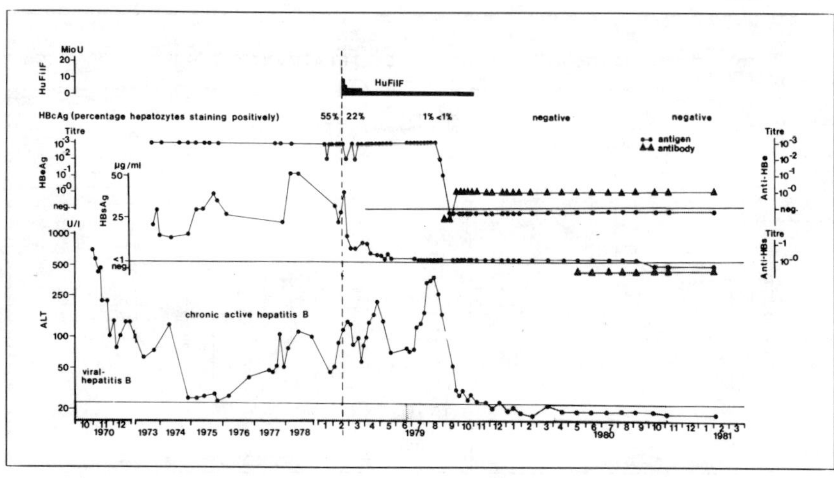

Fig. 3. Course of patient 1.

appearence of DNAP-activity and HBeAg from the serum as well as the normalization of liver-function tests in this patient cannot be regarded as a response to HuIFN-β treatment.

Follow-up of all patients, who completed post-treatment observations, was continued. In patient 1, HBsAG spontaneously disappeared from the serum 11 months after HuIFN-β treatment was stopped, thus showing that a type-2 response may turn into a type-1 response without any apparent exogenous antiviral procedures. Presence of anti-HBe and constantly normal liver-function tests in this patient were associated with a disappearance of HBcAg from the liver (fig. 3). On histological examination, features of chronic aggressive hepatitis were no longer detectable in 2 follow-up biopsies.

Patient 2 underwent immunosuppressive therapy 6 months after discontinuation of HuIFN-β treatment. Therapy was rapidly stopped in the same manner as it was done in patient 7 before participating in this study 2½ months after onset. It is particularly intriguing that this patient also responded with a complete suppression of HBV-infection including the disappearance of all markers indicating an ongoing HBV-infection, the normalization of liver-function tests, and the development of antibodies to HBs- and HBe-antigens.

So far no changes in the amount of HBsAg, HBeAg titers and liver-function tests in the controls were observed. Data regarding

DNAP-activity in these patients are not yet available, since sera are still undergoing investigation.

Discussion

Despite the fact that this study is not yet complete, there is some evidence that HuIFN-β, administered intravenously, exerts a suppressive effect on the indices of an ongoing HBV-infection, which is similar to that described in patients treated with HuIFN-α. 8 patients with CAHB revealed a significant decline of DNAP-activity in the serum, which is in accordance with findings of *Toshitsugu et al.*, who have observed a decrease of blood-DNAP in 3 women after intravenous injection of a total of 100 Mio U of HuIFN-β [16]. However, in all but one patient in this trial, DNAP-activity reappeared in the serum when lower doses of HuIFN-β were applied at longer intervals. Moreover, all but one patient also revealed persistent HBsAg, HBeAg, abnormal liver-function tests, and HBcAg in the liver tissue throughout a 15-month period of observation. A lasting suppression of HBV-markers, including the disappearance of HBsAg during long-term follow-up and a normalization of liver-function tests even upon cessation of therapy, was observed in only 1 individual.

Therefore we conclude that HuIFN-β, applied as single-agent treatment regimen, does not usually contribute to clinical improvement of the disease. It may, however, turn out to be a helpful adjuvant drug together with other antiviral procedures in the treatment of CAHB, since HuIFN-β exerts some temporary suppressive effect on HBV-replication. Our efforts are currently directed towards the search of a combination of antiviral treatment and stimulatory procedures on host-recovery responses, as they were observed in patient 7 during pretreatment observation and in patient 2 during post-treatment follow-up, which might achieve optimum therapeutic results.

References

1 Desmyter, J.; De Groote, J.; Desmet, V. J.; Billiau, A.; Ray, M. B.; Bradburne, A. F.; Edy, V. G.; De Somer, P.; Mortelmans, J.: Administration of human fibroblast interferon in chronic hepatitis B infection. Lancet *ii:* 645 – 647 (1976).

2 Dolen, J. G.; Carter, W. A.; Horoszewicz, J. S.; Vladutin, A. O.; Leibowitz, A. I.; Nolan, J. P.: Fibroblast interferon treatment of a patient with chronic active hepatitis. Am. J. Med. *67:* 127 – 131 (1979).

3 Dunnick, J. K.; Galasso, G. J.: Update on clinical trials with exogenous interferon. J. infect. Dis. *142:* 293 – 299 (1980).
4 Dunnick, J. K.; Galasso, G. J.: Clinical trials with exogenous interferon. J. infect. Dis. *139:* 109 – 123 (1979).
5 Edy, V. G.; Billiau, A.; De Somer, P.: Non-appearance of injected fibroblast interferon in circulation. Lancet *i:* 451 – 452 (1978).
6 Gerlich, W.; Thomssen, R.: Standardized detection of hepatitis B surface antigen: Determination of its serum concentration in weight units per volume. Devl Biol. *30:* 78 – 87 (1975).
7 Greenberg, H. B.; Pollard, R. B.; Lutwick, L. I.; Gregory, P. B.; Robinson, W. S.; Merigan, T. C.: Effect of human leukocyte interferon on hepatitis B virus infection in patients with chronic active hepatitis. New Engl. J. Med. *295:* 517 – 522 (1976).
8 Hill, D. A.; Walsh, S. H.; Purcell, R. H.: Failure to demonstrate circulating interferon during incubation period and acute stage of transfusion-associated hepatitis. Proc. Soc. exp. Biol. Med. *136:* 853 – 856 (1971).
9 Kaplan, P. M.; Greenman, R. L.; Gerin, J. L.; Purcell, R. H.; Robinson, W. S.: DNA-polymerase associated with human hepatitis-B-antigen. J. Virol. *12:* 995 – 1005 (1973).
10 Kingham, J. G. C.; Ganguly, N. K.; Shaari, Z. D.; Mendelson, R.; McGuire, M. J.; Holgate, S. J.; Cartwright, T.; Scott, G. M.; Richards, B. M.; Wright, R.: Treatment of HBsAg-positive chronic active hepatitis with human fibroblast interferon. Gut *19:* 91 – 94 (1978).
11 Merigan, T. C.; Robinson, W. S.: Antiviral therapy in HBV-infection. In: Vyas, Cohen, Schmid (eds.), Viral hepatitis, pp. 575 – 579 (Franklin Institute Press, Philadelphia 1978).
12 Merigan, T. C.: Interferon therapy in human viral infections and malignant disease. Conference on Clinical Potency of Interferon in Viral Diseases and Malignant Tumors, Oiso, Japan, December 1980.
13 Müller, R.; Vido, I.; Schmidt, F. W.: Rapid withdrawal of immunosuppressive therapy in chronic active hepatitis B. Lancet *i:* 1323 – 1324 (1981)
14 Taylor, P. E.; Zuckerman, A. J.: Non-production of interfering substances by serum from patients with infectious hepatitis. J. med. Microbiol. *1:* 217 – 222 (1968).
15 Tolentino, P.; Dianzani, F.; Zucca, M.; Giacchino, R. J.: Decreased interferon response by lymphocytes from children with chronic hepatitis. J. infect. Dis. *132:* 459 – 461 (1975).
16 Toshitsugu, O.; Hepatitis Research Committee: Effect of human leucocyte or fibroblast interferon on hepatitis B virus infection in patients with chronic hepatitis. Conference on Clinical Potency of Interferon in Viral Diseases and Malignant Tumors, Oiso, Japan, December 1980.
17 Weimar, W.; Heijtink, R. A.; Schalm, S. W.; Van Blankenstein, M.; Schellekens, H.; Masurel, N.; Edy, V. G.; Billiau, A.; De Somer, P.: Fibroblast interferon in HBsAg-positive chronic active hepatitis. Lancet *ii:* 1282 (1977).
18 Weimar, W.; Heijtink, R. A.; Ten Kate, F. J. P.; Schalm, S. W.; Masurel, N.; Schellekens, J.: Double-blind study of leukocyte interferon administration in chronic HBsAg-associated hepatitis. Lancet *i:* 336 – 338 (1980).
19 Wheelock, E. F.; Schenker, S.; Combes, B.: Absence of circulating interferon in patients with infectious and serum hepatitis. Proc. Soc. exp. Biol. Med. *128:* 251 – 253 (1968).

Prof. Dr. Rainer Müller, Abt. für Gastroenterologie und Hepatologie, Zentrum Innere Medizin, Med. Hochschule Hannover, Karl-Wiechert-Allee 9, D-3000 Hannover 61

Experience with Fibroblast-Derived Interferon as an Antitumor Agent[1]

D. Niethammer and J. Treuner

Abt. für pädiatrische Hämatologie, Universität Tübingen, FRG

Introduction

Strander et al. [1] have introduced leukocyte interferon (IFN-α) into clinical use as an adjuvant therapy in osteogenic sarcoma. This type of interferon is still used in most clinical trials by the group and other investigators. Only few reports on the use of fibroblast-derived interferon (IFN-β) exist [2–5]. In spite of its higher yield due to the superinduction, which is possible in fibroblasts but not in leukocytes, IFN-β is difficult to produce.

Nevertheless in Germany, the only available interferon for clinical use at present is IFN-β. The dramatic response seen in a boy with terminal nasopharyngeal carcinoma using this interferon [6] prompted us to treat other patients with IFN-β and to initiate a clinical trial in neuroblastoma stage IV [7]. The following paper deals with certain aspects of the clinical use of IFN-β as an antitumor agent in various forms of malignant diseases.

Interferon

The IFN-β, which we used, was prepared by Rentschler Co, Laupheim, Germany (supported by the German Ministry for Research and Technology). The specific activity varied from about 1 to 3×10^6 IU/mg protein. The interferon was delivered in liophilized

[1] Supported by a grant from the Deutsche Forschungsgemeinschaft (Forschergruppe Leukämieforschung, Tübingen)

Table I: Interferon plasma levels after different modes of application and various dosages

Time (min)	subc.	i.m.	2.4×10^6 IU/m²				4.8×10^6 IU/m⁶	9.6×10^6 IU/m²
			i.v. push	i.v. 30 min	i.v. 60 min	i.v. 240 min	i.v. 30 min	i.v. 30 min
5	n.d.	n.d.	128	32	8	8	96	384
10	0	0	96	64	24	n.d.	192	384
15	n.d.	n.d.	32	96	48	n.d.	192	384
30	0	0	24	128	48	n.d.	32	n.d.
45	n.d.	n.d.	12	32	n.d.	n.d.	12	128
60	0	0	0	24	48	8	44	64
90	n.d.	n.d.	n.d.	8	48	n.d.	44	64
120	0	0	n.d.	8	n.d.	10	32	32
180	n.d.	n.d.	n.d.	n.d.	n.d.	n.d.	n.d.	32
360	0	0	n.d.	0	n.d.	12	n.d.	n.d.

form and stored at −20°C. It was dissolved in physiological saline immediately before injection. Interferon concentrations were determined by two different cytopathic effect inhibition assays [8, 9].

Pharmacokinetic Properties

The first question we asked ourselves was what the best route and time of administration of IFN-β would be [10]. Table I summarizes the interferon plasma levels obtained from different modes of application and various dosages of IFN-β in children. In contrast to IFN-α, detectable serum levels could only be achieved after i. v. injections. These data confirm clinical and experimental observations in animals [11, 12]. It has been demonstrated that human IFN-β can only be traced in extremely low amounts when not administered intravenously into rabbits and that it cannot be discovered at all in most organs. This might be due to absorption of IFN-β in the soft tissue or even to inactivation at the site of injection [12].

Intravenous push injections of IFN-β only led to short-lasting serum levels which could be prolonged when infusions over 30 min or even several hours were used. But as expected, lower peak levels were obtained at the same time. The peak levels, achieved under identical conditions in different children, correlated well with the body surface of the children and the amount infused [10].

Our data suggest that long-term infusions of IFN-β, lasting at least 12 h, would be necessary to achieve serum levels which are comparable to those seen after i.m. injections of IFN-α. As a result, much larger quantities of IFN-β would have to be used.

As yet it is not known what significance the time of persistance and the achieved level of IFN in the plasma may have on its effectiveness as an antitumor agent. In vitro studies have suggested that the effect of IFN on the reduction of cell growth is identical when IFN is present between 2 and 24 h [13]. On the other hand, numerous experiments have shown that the antiproliferative action of IFN is dose-dependent. This suggests that the achieved peak serum level might be more important than the time period during which IFN is present.

Our data, obtained from children, show that IFN-β should be administered intravenously to achieve reasonable serum levels. Nevertheless, there is evidence that the amount of natural-killer cells increase even after i.m. injection of IFN-β [14] suggesting a positive effect after all. On the other hand – in our opinion – the increase of natural-killer cell activity, induced by interferon, does not prove any antitumor activity of IFN and it is probably induced by very small amounts of IFN. In clinical studies, the response of the natural-killer cells does not correlate with that of the tumor. For our clinical trials we decided that infusions lasting 30 min would be a good compromise between the two parameters: the peak level and the length of measurable IFN concentrations. We have used this mode of application in the meantime even on an outpatient basis.

Antibodies against IFN-β

The production of heterologous antibodies has been induced in animals against human interferons and it was demonstrated that the antigenicity of IFN-α and IFN-β is different, so that antibodies against the one IFN did not react with the other [15]. Additional studies have shown that IFNs are not antigenic in a homologous system.

Nevertheless, we decided to perform regular controls of the achieved serum levels in children, who were treated over longer periods with IFN-β. To our surprise, we found in one patient with naso-

Table II. Summary of the results of some of the experiments which suggest the presence of neutralizing antibodies in the patient's cells [16]

Interferon	Additions to the assay	Inhibition of IFN activity by patient's pre-treatment serum
IFN-β (Rentschler)	0	0
		Inhibition of IFN-activity by patient's post-treatment serum
IFN-β (Rentschler)	0	+
IFN-β (NIH)	0	+
IFN-β (Rentschler)	fetal calf serum	+
IFN-α (Cantell)	0	0
IFN-α (Cantell)	[1]FS4-cell preparation	0

[1] FS4-cells are the foreskin fibroblasts from which the IFN-β (Rentschler) is produced.

pharyngeal carcinoma, who had successfully been treated with IFN-β [6], that after 6 months no interferon levels could be detected any more after the infusion of 4×10^6 IU. This was confirmed by several controls and we decided to analyze the serum for neutralizing antibodies against IFN-β [16]. It could be demonstrated that there was indeed IFN-neutralizing activity present in the serum which inhibited IFN-β but not IFN-α (table II). In addition we could demonstrate that in the patient's serum a highly spontaneous IFN titer was detectable during an acute virus infection, which was most likely due to the production of IFN-α. The result after the addition of FS4-cell preparation ruled out the possibility that the presence of antibodies against antigens of the FS4-cell preparation other than IFN-β coprecipitated with IFN to produce a reaction which was erroneously interpreted as IFN-β neutralization. However, we cannot exclude the possibility that the antibody observed was produced against a complex of IFN-β + FS4-protein which could be a result of the method of purification. At least, the IFN-β from NIH was inhibited to the same extent suggesting that it might have been an anti-IFN-β. In further experiments we could demonstrate that the IFN-β-neutralizing activity was in fact due to an IgG-antibody [16]. It was shown that the anti-IFN-β activity remained in a purified IgG-fraction. Immunodiffusion showed that there was no IgA or IgM. Immunoelectrophoresis against rabbit anti-human serum protein revealed only one component in the IgG preparation.

This is the first demonstration of homologous antibodies against IFN and of antibodies produced in a human being. A number of other patients have been treated with the same IFN over longer periods of time but IFN-neutralizing activity was never detected in their serum [10].

There are several possible explanations for the production of these antibodies: (a) It is possible that the IFN-β-molecule is altered by the purification in a way that it becomes antigenic; (b) The patient's cells lack the genes for IFN-β; (c) There exist different IFN-βs in man with different antigenicity and the patient might have had a rare type. Recently, another patient with anti-IFN-β antibodies was supposedly discovered in Canada [17].

The fact that no antibodies have been detected against IFN-α, as yet, might be explained in different ways: (a) Many patients who were treated with IFN-α had never been tested for antibodies; (b) More than ten different IFN-αs have been demonstrated in man and the used preparations are mixtures of them. It is possible that the antigenicity of these interferons differ so that antibodies are produced only against one of them. In this case it would be difficult to detect the antibodies by testing for neutralizing activity.

The future will have to show how frequent the production of antibodies is during the treatment with IFN and the use of monoclonal interferons might help to explain the true cause of this phenomenon.

Antitumor Effect of IFN-β

The true value of IFN is still not known at present time. This is true for both kinds of IFN, IFN-α as well as IFN-β. Dramatic responses like that seen by us in a boy suffering from an end-stage nasopharyngeal carcinoma [6] might lead to an overestimation of the potentials of IFN. In addition to this patient, we have treated five children with nasopharyngeal carcinoma [18]. In 2 of them, whose tumors were rather similar to that of the first boy, the increase of the rapidly growing tumors was stopped for 4 and 8 months but no regression of the tumors could be demonstrated. One patient received interferon as an initial treatment. This was stopped after 9 days because of severe side effects, rendering this patient unevaluable. No effect at all could be observed in 2 children with extensive metastatic lesions. Nasopharyngeal carcinoma is a rare tumor in children. It might be different from the nasopharyngeal carcinoma, which is a common cause of death in adults coming from Southern China, but the morphology and the relationship to the Epstein-Barr virus is identical for both of them. A possible virus induction of this tumor makes it more likely that IFN might act inhibitory in this tumor.

At present time studies have been started in various parts of China to prove or disprove a positive effect of IFN on this tumor. The studies of our six children showed a positive effect in half of them. In the near future it will have to be shown how active IFN is as a single agent in this disease. It might be much better to use it in a prophylactic way to prevent relapses instead of treating the advanced disease.

Various patients with other tumors have been treated with IFN-β without clear evidence of a response. These include spindle-cell sarcoma, osteogeneic sarcoma with metastatic lesions, acute leukemia (ALL and AML), colon carcinoma, malignant melanoma, carcinoid, and others. They were all single cases which have been treated outside of a protocol; with various dosages, administration schedules, and differing lengths of therapy.

In addition, and more important, clinical trials have been started for neuroblastoma stage IV, gastric cancer, osteogenic sarcoma, low-grade malignant lymphoma in adults, and myeloma. For the latter there is some evidence that IFN-β, like IFN-α, can induce a positive response in some patients [19]. The design for the therapeutical trial of neuroblastoma stage IV will be discussed during this meeting [7] and has already been presented elsewhere [20]. The design of this study, like that of the osteogenic sarcoma trial, uses chemotherapy to reduce the tumor mass. IFN is added later to the chemotherapy and, in the case of neuroblastoma, it is continued after the end of chemotherapy. In contrast, the trial for gastric cancer is a randomized adjuvant IFN therapy after surgery. Only those cases are included where the tumor is thought to be resected completely.

The results obtained with IFN-β as an antitumor agent are still not very clear. Two to three years will be necessary to complete most of the clinical trials before anything can be said. There is no doubt that the following questions cannot be answered at present time.

(1) Does IFN-β act as an antitumor agent in vivo so that it can be used as a therapeutic factor?

(2) If the clinical trials do not show a positive effect of IFN-β, is this due to the ineffectiveness of IFN-β or is it due to mistakes in the design of the trial (dose, schedule, combination with chemotherapy, etc.)?

Much work will have to be done and patience will be necessary until we know the true value of IFN-β as well that of the other interferons.

References

1 Strander, H.; Cantell, K.; Carlstrom, G.; Jakobsson, P. A.: Clinical and laboratory investigations on man; Systemic administration of potent interferon to man. J. natn. Cancer Inst. *51:*733 (1973).

2 Horoszewicz, J. S.; Leong, S. S.; Ito, M.; Buffet, R.; Karakousis, C.; Holyoke, E.; Job, I.; Carter, W. A.: Human Fibroblast Interferon in Human Neoplasia: Clinical and Laboratory Study. Cancer Treatm. (11) *62:*1899 (1978).

3 Nemoto, T.; Carter, W. A.; Dolen, J. G.; Holyoke, D.; Horoszewicz, J. S.: Human interferons and intralesional therapy of melanoma and breast carcinoma. Am. Assoc. Cancer Res. *20:*246 (1979).

4 McPherson, T. A.; Tan, Y. H.: Phase-I pharmacotoxicology study of human fibroblast interferon in human cancers. J. natn. Cancer Inst. (1) *65:*75 (1980).

5 Dunnick, J. K.; Galasso, G. J.: Clinical Trials with Exogenous Interferon: Summary of a Meeting. J. infect. Dis. *139:*109 (1979).

6 Treuner, J.; Niethammer, D.; Dannecker, G.; Hagmann, R.; Neef, V.; Hofschneider, P. H.: Successful treatment of nasopharyngeal carcinoma with interferon. Lancet *i:*817 (1980).

7 Lampert, F.; Berthold, F.; Treuner, J.; Niethammer, D.: Therapeutical trial for neuroblastoma stage IV (GPO-Study NBL-79). This book, pp. 114.

8 Wagner, R. R.: Biological studies of interferon suppression of cellular infection with eastern equine encephalomyelitis virus. Virology *13:*323 (1961).

9 Dake, H.; Degre, M.: A micro assay for mouse and human interferon. Acta. pathol. microbiol. scand. *380:*863 (1972).

10 Treuner, J.; Dannecker, G.; Joester, K.-E.; Hettinger, A.; Niethammer, D.: Pharmacological aspects of clinical stage I/II trials with human fibroblast interferon in children. Int. J. Interferon Res. *3:*373 (1981).

11 Carter, W. A.; Horoszewicz, J.: Production, purification, and clinical application of human fibroblast interferon. Pharmacol. Ther. *8:*359 (1980).

12 Hanley, D. F.; Wiranowska-Stewart, M.; Stewart, W. E., II: Pharmacology of interferons. I: Pharmacological distinctions between human leukocyte- and fibroblast interferons. Int. J. Immunopharmac. *1:*219 (1979).

13 Pfeffer, L. M.: Interferon effects on the growth and division of human fibroblasts. Exp. Cell Res. *121:*111 (1979).

14 Billiau, A.: Personal communication.

15 Levy-König, R. E.; Golgner, R. R.; Paucker, K.: Immunology of interferons. Heterospecific activities of human interferons and their neutralization by antibody. J. Immun. *104:*791 (1970).

16 Vallbracht, A.; Treuner, J.; Flehmig, B.; Joester, K.-E.; Niethammer, D.: Interferon-neutralizing antibodies in a patient treated with human fibroblast interferon. Nature *289:*496 (1981).

17 Berthold, W.: Personal communication

18 Treuner, J.; Niethammer, D.; Dannecker, G.; Jobke, A.; Aldenhoff, P.; Kremens, B.; Nessler, G.; Bömer, H.: Treatment of nasopharyngeal carcinoma in children with fibroblast interferon. XII. International Symposium Nasopharyngeal Carci-

noma. Basis Research as Applied to Diagnosis and Therapy, Düsseldorf, October 1980 (in press).

19 Wilms, K.: Personal communication

20 Berthold, F.; Treuner, J.; Niethammer, D.; Lampert, F.: Neuroblastomstudie NBL 79 der Gesellschaft für pädiatrische Onkologie, Zwischenbericht nach 1 Jahr. Ergebnisse der pädiatrischen Onkologie (in press).

Prof. Dr. D. Niethammer, Universitäts-Kinderklinik, Abt. Hämatologie, D-7400 Tübingen

Therapeutical Trial for Neuroblastoma Stage IV

(GPO-Study NBL-79)[1]

F. Lampert, F. Berthold, J. Treuner, D. Niethammer

Kinderkliniken der Universitäten Gießen und Tübingen, FRG

Introduction

Neuroblastoma is the most common solid tumor in children and comprises about 8% of all malignant diseases in childhood. A little over 100 new patients per year are expected in West Germany. The majority of patients is less than 3 years old at diagnosis. Up to 70% of patients have disseminated tumor at diagnosis, affecting mainly bone marrow and bones. Prognosis is related to age and stage of the disease [1]. Treatment, thus, is different from patient to patient and must be adjusted to the clinical stage (table I). Over 1-year-old children with stage-IV neuroblastoma at diagnosis have less than 5% chance of survival despite all kinds of chemotherapy tried in the past 15 years [2]. These patients are studied in a nation-wide chemotherapy-interferon trial by the GPO (German Pediatric Oncology) group.

Patients

Until 1 March 1981, a total of 80 children with neuroblastoma stage-IV disease, diagnosed since 1979, have been registered from 30 hospitals of the Federal Republic of Germany. 15 children were under 1 year of age. 13 patients were not available for the protocol because of other previous therapies. Thus, 52 patients could enter the chemotherapy-interferon study GPO-NBL_{79} and 26 were randomized for interferon after the first 3 cycles of chemotherapy.

[1] Supported by the Bundesministerium für Forschung und Technologie, Bonn

Table I. Neuroblastoma: Clinical stages and treatment

Stage		Therapy
I	Localized tumor completely resected	Surgery
II	Localized tumor residual microscopic tumor	Surgery ± Radiotherapy
III	Localized or regional tumor incompletely resected	Surgery Chemotherapy (ACVD) ± "Second look" ± Radiotherapy
IV	Disseminated tumor distant metastases	Chemotherapy (ACVD) ± Interferon ± Surgery ± Radiotherapy

A = Adriamycin; C = Cyclophosphamide; V = Vincristine; D = Dacarbazin

Table II. Disseminated neuroblastoma: Chemotherapy - GPO-Protocol NBL-79

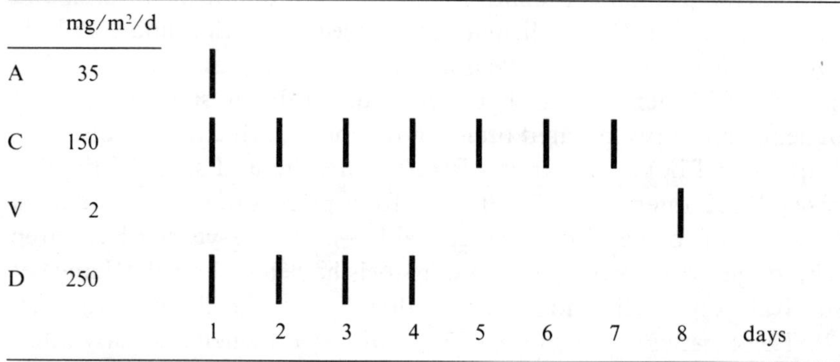

	mg/m²/d	1	2	3	4	5	6	7	8 days
A	35	|							
C	150	|	|	|	|	|	|	|	
V	2								|
D	250	|	|	|	|				

Repeat every 3 weeks for a total of 8 cycles;
omit V + D after 3rd cycle;
random. for ± interferon after 3rd cycle

Therapy Design

Chemotherapy for disseminated neuroblastoma is a combination of 4 drugs, namely adriamycin, cyclophosphamide, vincristine, DTIC or dacarbazin, which as single agents, have previously shown action against neuroblastoma cells. Therapy is applied in cycles (table II), each lasting for 8 days and repeated every 3 weeks if leukocytes of the patients have recovered above 2000/µl. After the 3rd cycle, vincris-

Table III. Disseminated neuroblastoma: Fibroblast interferon – addition to chemotherapy

10^5 U/KG I.V. 30 MIN INFUSION

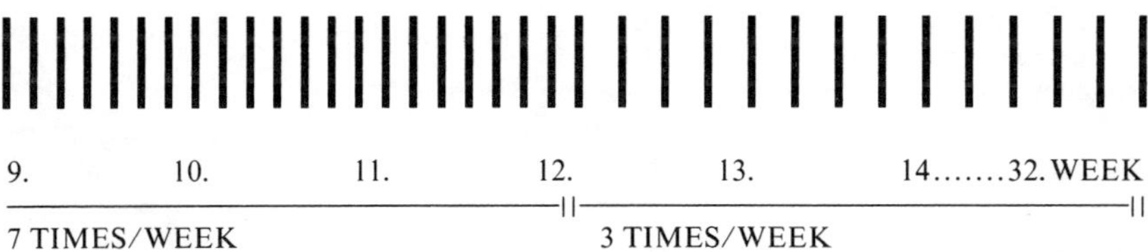

tine and DTIC are omitted. A total of 8 cycles is given over a period of 6 months. The most active part of the chemotherapy is probably the 1 week of cyclophosphamide (150 mg/m^2/day $\times$ 7). The patients were randomized to receive either Yes or No interferon after the 3rd cycle or 9th week (table III). When an inoperable primary tumor regresses due to chemotherapy treatment, a second-look operation with tumor removal is carried out. Interferon in an approximate dose of 10^5 units per kg body weight is given as a 30 min infusion daily the first 3 weeks, then 3 times per week the following 32 weeks. Interferon can be given on the same day as chemotherapy although several hours between chemotherapy and interferon injections is advised.

Preliminary Results

After 9 weeks of chemotherapy, 79% of the patients responded favorably. 37% attained a complete (disappearance of tumor masses and all tumor cells were microscopically undetectable in bone marrow) and 42% a partial remission.

There were fewer relapses (5/26) and deaths (1/26) in the group randomized for additional interferon therapy compared to the group which received chemotherapy only: 9/26 relapses and 6/26 dead (table IV).

Off therapy and living in complete continuous remission are 7 patients (longest observation time being 24 months) in the interferon group versus only 1 patient (16 months) in the chemotherapy only group.

A proper evaluation of the additional effect of interferon, however, will only be possible in another year when more than 100 pa-

Table IV. Disseminated neuroblastoma: GPO-study NBL-79 (1 March 1981)

Enter study (from 30 hospitals)		80 Patients
Under 1 year		15
Evaluable for protocol		52
Randomized for	+ IF	26
	− IF	26
Relapses	+ IF	5 (1 dead)
	− IF	9 (6 dead)
Off therapy in CCR	+ IF	7
	− IF	1

IF = Fibroblast Interferon; CCR = Complete Continuous Remission

tients have been studied and released from therapy. The only side effect of interferon was hyperpyrexia after initial injections.

Life-table analysis as of 1 August 1981 revealed a survival rate of 0.32 for the interferon group vs. 0.22 for the non-interferon group. The difference, however, is not statistically significant. No difference was observed for the remission rate between the two groups.

References

1 Evans, A. E.: Staging and treatment of neuroblastoma. Cancer *45:* 1799–1802 (1980).

2 Finklestein, J. Z.; Klemperer, M. R.; Evans, A.; Bernstein, I.; Leikin, S.; McCreadie, S.; Grosfeld, J.; Hittle, R.; Weiner, J.; Sather, H.; Hammond, D.: Multiagent Chemotherapy for Children with Metastatic Neuroblastoma: A Report from Children's Cancer Study Group. Med. Pediat. Oncol. *6:* 179–188 (1979).

Prof. Dr. Fritz Lampert, Universitäts-Kinderpoliklinik, D-6300 Gießen

Interferon in Non-Hodgkin-Lymphoma of Low Malignancy

D. Huhn[1], *U. Fink*[2], *H. Theml*[3], *W. Siegert*[1], *G. Riethmüller*[4], *W. Wilmanns*[1]

[1] Medizinische Klinik III, Klinikum Großhadern, Universität München, FRG
[2] Klinikum Rechts der Isar der Techn. Universität München, FRG
[3] Städtisches Krankenhaus München-Schwabing, FRG
[4] Immunologisches Institut der Universität München, FRG

Until March 1981 results had been published of about 60 lymphoma patients treated with interferon (IFN). As indicated in table I, response to treatment was observed in about 50% of patients, most of whom had been pretreated with cytostatics and/or irradiation and suffered from advanced lymphoma manifestation. In non-Hodgkin-lymphoma (NHL), including chronic lymphatic leukemia (CLL), complete remission (CR) was obtained in 2, and partial response (PR) in 11 of 23 patients treated with IFN. CR was seen in NHL of nodular type, whilst in NHL of non-favorable histology (diffuse histiocytic) no response was attained. In nearly all cases leukocyte IFN (IFN-α) was used. Side effects were fever in almost all cases, and granulocytopenia and thrombocytopenia in some patients; cytopenia was never so severe as to cause interruption of treatment.

A clinical trial to test the effectiveness and the side effects of IFN in NHL of low malignancy therefore seems legitimate, and a pilot study was started in three clinical institutions in Munich. The setting of this study will be introduced briefly in the following.

Patients and Methods

Patients may enter the study when the following criteria are met:

(1) Diagnosis of NHL of low malignancy according to *Kiel* classification [4] as indicated in table II.

(2) Stage III and IV (according to *Rai* classification, [15]) in CCL,

Table I: Results of IFN therapy in malignant lymphoma

Lymphoma	References	IFN	No. of pat.	Response to therapy CR	PR	LPR SD	PD
M. Hodgkin	3	α	1		1		
	5	α/β	4	1	3		
Plasmocytoma	1	α	3		3		
	10	α	4		4		
	7	α	10	1	2	3	4
	12	β	10		3		7
ALL	2	α	4			4	
	8	α	2		2		
CLL	7	α	4		1	1	2
	12	α	9		6		3
NHL							
– nodular	11	α	3		3		
	7	α	6	2	1		3
– diff. hist.	11	α	3				3
	7	α	1			1	
Total			64	4	29	9	22

Table II. Subtypes of NHL of low malignancy according to *Kiel*-classification

Chronic lymphatic leukemia (CLL)
- B- or T-subtype
- prolymphocytic (PCLL)

Immunocytoma (IC)
Centrocytoma (CC)
Centroblastic-centrocytic lymphoma (CBCC)

and stage IV (according to *Ann Arbor*) in the remaining subtypes of low malignant NHL.

(3) Pretreatment with cytostatics, corticosteroids, or irradiation may have been performed, but a treatment-free interval of 4 weeks before start with IFN was obligatory.

(4) Voluntary consent of informed patients to be treated.

Clinical investigations to determine the stage of the disease and the response to therapy are as follows:

(1) Measurement of representative lymphomas in all accessible re-

gions and calculation of an index given by the sum of the products of diameters (width times length); x-ray of the chest, when questionable supplemented by tomography, and measurement of the area of enlarged hilar lymphomas using a semi-automatic analysing system (MOP Digiplan, KONTRON); abdominal computerized tomography (Dr. B. Sommer, Munich), and measurement of lymphoma area in representative tomographs as indicated above.

(2) When unequivocal palpation of the spleen is not possible, its size is measured by scintigraphy.

(3) Scintigraphy of the skeleton and roentgenography of questionable lesions.

(4) Bone-marrow histology and quantification of lymphoma-involved areas (Dr. R. Bartl, Munich).

(5) Liver histology when stage IV cannot be verified otherwise.

(6) Routine laboratory tests are complemented with determination of polyclonal and of monoclonal immunoglobulins; cytochemistry and membrane-marker tests of blood or bone-marrow cells or of lymph-node imprints to determine the subtype of lymphoma and the extent of leukemic manifestation with the best possible accuracy (Dr. E. Thiel, Munich).

In addition, CFU-C of bone-marrow cells (Dr. L. Böning, Munich), and NK activity (Dr. Kaudewitz, Munich) were investigated.

Criteria for response are modifications of those suggested by the International Union Against Cancer and modified according to *Gutterman* [7].

Complete remission (CR) indicates disappearance of all known disease.

Partial remission (PR) is at least a 50% decrease of measurable lesions (lymphoma index, area of hilar or abdominal lymphoma, spleen size, bone-marrow infiltration, amount of monoclonal immunoglobulin and of lymphoma cells in the blood) and objective improvement in evaluable, but nonmeasurable lesions. No lesion may have progressed nor any new lesions appeared.

Less than partial remissions (LPR) indicates a 25% to 50% decrease in measurable lesions.

Stable disease (SD) is defined as lesions which remained unchanged for at least 8 weeks, and a less than 25% decrease or increase in the size of measurable lesions.

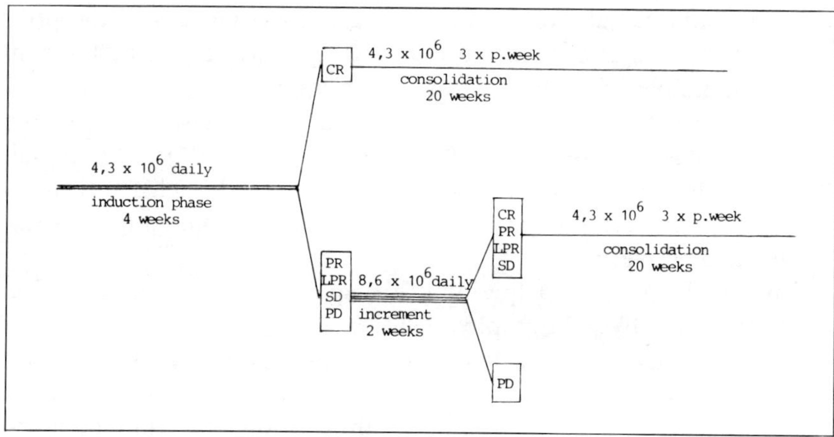

Figure 1: Application of IFN in NHL of low malignancy.

Progressive disease (PD) is a greater than or equal to 25% increase in size of any lesions, or appearance of new lesions, or a mixed progressive and regressive response.

Source of IFN and schedule for dose and application. Fibroblast IFN (IFN-β) used for our pilot study is made available by Dr. Rentschler, Laupheim (West Germany). Therapy is started with 4.3×10^6. U of IFN given daily as a 30-min infusion for 4 weeks (fig. 1). In case of PR, LPR, SD, and PD the dose of IFN is increased (after 4 weeks of treatment) to 8.6×10^6 U daily for another 2 weeks. If life-threatening lymphoma progression occurs during the first 4 weeks of treatment, the dose may be doubled earlier. When CR is obtained after 4 weeks of treatment, and in case of CR, PR, LPR, of SD after dose increment, "consolidation" is started with 4.3×10^6 U of IFN three times a week for another 20 weeks. In case of PD no consolidation treatment is given. As soon as criteria for PD evolve during consolidation therapy, IFN is stopped.

Results

Preliminary results of the pilot study testing effectiveness of IFN-β in NHL of low malignancy are as follows. In March 1981 results of induction and increment phase were evaluable in 7 patients (table

Table III: Results of IFN-β treatment in 7 patients. Abbreviations of diagnoses see table II.
ϟ = irradiation; Chl = chlorambucil, P = prednisolone, C = cyclophosphamide, O = vincristine, Pr = procarbazine

Age Diagnosis	Time Diagnosis – IFN (months)	Pre-treatment	Stage before IFN	Result after induction and increment	> 50% Fall of	
					Granulocytes	Platelets
72 ♀ PCLL	6	ϟ Chl P	IV A (Rai)	PD	0	0
45 ♂ IC	84	ϟ Chl P	IV A	SD	↓	0
42 ♂ IC	24	Chl P	IV A	SD (PD after 1 month of consolidation)	After induct. ↓ After increm. 0	0
43 ♂ IC	60	ϟ P	IV A	PD	0	0
60 ♂ CC	36	Chl P CoPrP	IV A	PD	0	0
32 ♂ CBCC	42	COP ϟ	IV A	PD	0	0
66 ♀ CBCC	36	ϟ COP	IV A	SD	0	0

III). Mean age of the patients was 51 years, mean time from diagnosis to start of IFN treatment 41 months, all patients were stages IV A. All patients had been pretreated, in most cases with irradiation and with either chlorambucil and prednisolone or with a mixture of cyclophosphamide, vincristine, and prednisolone. According to measurable lymph nodes, spleen, or leukemic cells in the blood, disease was progressive after induction and increment in 5 patients (in one case not before 1 month of consolidation therapy), and stable in 2 patients.

Side effects were fever with peaks between 38° and 39°C in all patients. A decrease in granulocytes of more than 50% compared with pretreatment values occurred in 1 patient only and was reversible during IFN treatment in a second one. Platelets remained fairly stable. Serious side effects have not been observed.

Discussion

NHL of low malignancy show generalization early during the course of the disease. When generalization has occurred, curative treatment by irradiation or cytostatics is no longer within reach [4]. The spontaneous course of the disease is usually characterized by a rather slow, but constant progression of lymphoma manifestation [16]. The 50% survival probability is about 72 months [4]. In a retrospective analysis of 209 cases of NHL and during an observation period of 28 years, a spontaneous regression of tumor manifestations was observed in 20 patients; regression in most cases was incomplete and of limited duration [6]. Effectiveness of IFN in our pilot study, therefore, was evaluated in comparison with the course of the disease before and after IFN treatment in an individual patient.

In NHL, especially in CLL and in IC, the progression of the disease may be rather slow, requiring no immediate specific therapy. When a specific therapy seems necessary, efficacy of cytostatics and prednisolone at the first trial is fairly certain, resulting in remissions in more than 50% of patients [13, 14] and in stabilization of disease parameters in almost all of the remaining patients. In addition to using therapy with IFN, CR was achieved according to literature (table I) in patients who had been heavily pretreated and suffered from extended disease. It did not seem justified, therefore, to restrict IFN application to patients who had not been treated before.

The exact histological diagnosis of subtypes of NHL is often difficult, and transitions from one subtype to another may be observed during the course of the disease. All subtypes of NHL of low malignancy, therefore, were included in our study; and a new biopsy and confirmation of histological diagnosis were required in cases where the last histological diagnosis were not within 6 months before IFN. Our pilot study, therefore, included all subtypes of NHL of low malignancy; and stratification of final results according to histological subtype may be performed.

Preliminary therapeutic results do not as yet appear very promising, but the results of a definitive evaluation remain to be seen.

References

1 Aare, In: Dunnick, Galasso, Clinical trials with exogenous interferon: Summary of a meeting. J. infect. Dis. *139:* 109–123 (1979).

2 Åhlström, L.; Dohlwitz, A.; Strander, H.; Carlström, G.; Cantell, K.: Interferon in acute leukemia in children. Lancet *i:* 166–167 (1974).

3 Blomgren, H.; Cantell, K.; Johansson, B.; Lagergren, C.; Ringborg, U.; Strander, H.: Interferon therapy in Hodgkin's disease. Acta med. scand. *199:* 527–532 (1976).

4 Brittinger, G.; Schmalhorst, U.; Bartels, H.; Brücher, H.; Common, H.; Dühmke, E.; Fülle, H. H.; Gunzer, U.; Huhn, D.; König, E.; Lennert, K.; Leopold, H.; Meusers, P.; Nowicki, L.; Pralle, H.; Stacher, A.; Theml, H.: Clinical relevance of the Kiel classification of non-Hodgkin lymphomas: Preliminary results of a prospective multicentric study. In: Tagnon, Staquet, (eds.), Controversies in Cancer, pp. 175–187 (Masson Publ., Paris 1979).

5 Emödi, G. In: Dunnick, Galasso, Clinical trials with exogenous interferon: Summary of a meeting. J. infect. Dis. *139:* 109–123 (1979).

6 Gattiker, H. H.; Wiltshaw, E.; Galton, D. A. G.: Spontaneous regression in non-Hodgkin's lymphoma. Cancer *45:* 2627–2632 (1980).

7 Gutterman, J. U.; Blumenschein, G. R.; Alexanian, R.; Yap, H. Y.; Buzdar, A. U.; Cabanillas, F.; Hortobagyi, G. N.; Hersh, E. M.; Rasmussen, S. L.; Harmon, M.; Kramer, M.; Pestka, S.: Leukocyte interferon-induced tumor regression in human metastatic breast cancer, multiple myeloma, and malignant lymphoma. Ann. intern. Med. *93:* 399–406 (1980).

8 Hill, N. O.; Loeb, E.; Pardue, A.; Kahn, A.; Dorn, G. L.; Comparini, S.; Hill, J. M.: Leukocyte interferon production and its effectiveness in acute lymphatic leukemia. J. clin. Hemat. Oncol. *8:* 66 (1978).

9 Huhn, D.; Thiel, E.; Rodt, H.; Theml, H.: Prolymphocytic leukemia. Klin. Wschr. *56:* 709–714 (1978).

10 Mellstedt, H.; Ahre, A.; Björkholm, M.; Holm, G.; Johansson, B.; Strander, H.: Interferon therapy in myelomatosis. Lancet *i:* 245–247 (1979).

11 Merigan, T. C.; Sikora, K.; Breeden, J. H.; Levy, R.; Rosenberg, S. A.: Preliminary observations on the effect of human leukocyte interferon in non-Hodgkin's lymphoma. New Engl. J. Med. *299:* 1449–1453 (1978).

12 Misset, J. L.; Gounter, A.; Mathé, G.: Clinical and immunological experience of interferon in B-cell malignancies. European Society of Medical Oncology, 6th Annual Meeting (Nice, December 1980).

13 Portlock, C. S.; Rosenberg, S. A.; Glatstein, E.; Kaplan, H. S.: Treatment of advanced non-Hodgkin's lymphomas with favorable histologies: Preliminary results of a prospective trial. Blood *47;* 747–756 (1976).

14 Portlock, C. S.; Rosenberg, S. A.: No initial therapy for stage III and IV non-Hodgkin's lymphomas of favorable histologic types. Ann. intern. Med. *90:* 10–13 (1979).

15 Rai, K. P.; Sawitsky, A.; Cronkite, E. P.; Chanana, A. D.; Levy, R. N.; Pasternack, B. S.: Clinical staging of chronic lymphocytic leukemia. Blood *46:* 219–234 (1975).

16 Theml, H.; Rastetter, J.: Chronische lymphatische Leukämie: Klinische Phänomene als Ausdruck pathomechanischer Prozesse. Tempo Medical *3:* 12–19 (1978).

Prof. Dr. Huhn, Med. Klinik III, Klinikum Großhadern, Marchioninistr. 15, D-8000 München 70

Randomized Controlled Study to Examine the Effectiveness of Fibroblast Interferon as an Adjuvant Therapy in Gastric Carcinoma Operated for Cure

Ch. Herfarth, P. Schlag, W. Schreml

Department für Chirurgie, Universität Ulm, FRG

Since there are as yet no certified results on the effectiveness and the mechanism of action of interferon in the treatment of malignant tumors, an examination of the presumed antitumor properties of this substance is necessary [1]. In the beginning these investigations should be directed towards certain signal tumors whose model character would permit an appropriate transferability of the results obtained.

There are several reasons for choosing the gastric carcinoma as an appropriate signal tumor (fig. 1). Due to its very uniform and short course, therapeutic results on a standardized basis can be compared very quickly [3]. The therapeutic results obtained here can be carried over to the treatment of other gastro-intestinal carcinomas if the indications are suitable. The lack of any demonstrable effectiveness of interferon in gastric cancer would, therefore, indicate that this substance does not possess a general principle of action. One could then conclude that the other frequently occurring tumors of the intestinal tract, which are marked by their resistance to systemic therapeutic measures, are also not suitable for treatment with interferon. Conversely, the demonstration of interferon effectiveness in gastric cancer could signify a possible successful therapeutic concept for the large group of intestinal adenocarcinomas, which again would justify further investigations along this route (table I).

Inhibitory effects on the clonal tumor cell growth of gastric-cancer cells in vitro supplied indications for a cytotoxic action of interferon on this tumor [4]. Since, however, the antitumor mechanism of interferon action is thought to be primarily based on an immunomod-

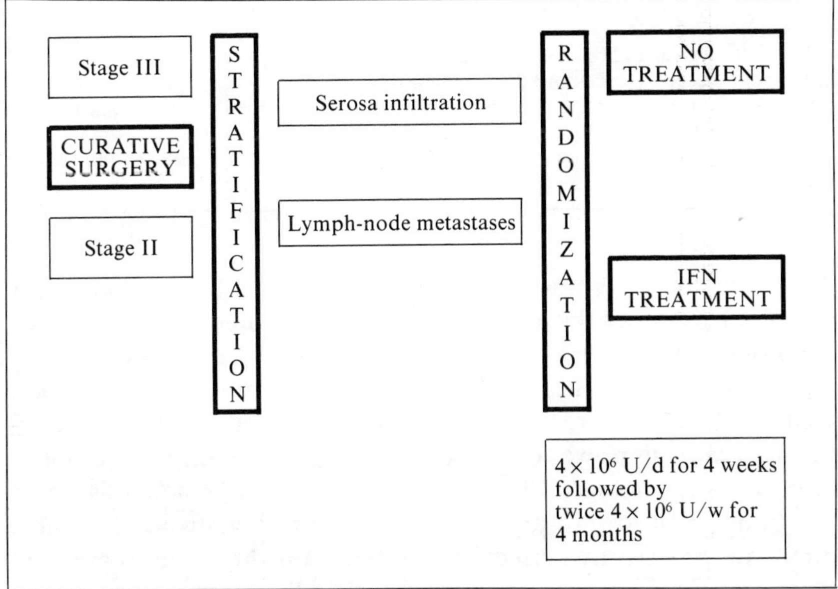

Figure 1. Adjuvant interferon trial in gastric cancer.

ulating principle [2], the use of this substance appears to be most promising under adjuvant therapy conditions.

Under these considerations we accordingly planned a controlled randomized adjuvant interferon study (fig. 1). All gastric-cancer patients with a tumor stage II or III, operated for potential cure, were included in the protocol. After stratifying the patients according to lymph-node involvement and serosa penetration, the patients were randomly divided into a control and a therapy group. Due to the as yet unknown effectiveness of interferon, the use of a control group is necessary and ethically justified in the case of gastric cancer, since there are no other effective adjuvant therapy modalities available for this tumor to date [3]. Interferon therapy begins between the 7th and

Table I. Rationale for interferon trials in gastric cancer

1. 'Marker'-tumor for gastro-intestinal carcinomas
2. Homogeneous, short course of the disease
3. No other effective adjuvant therapy available
4. Proven cytotoxicity of IFN in gastric cancer stem cells

Table II. Aim of the adjuvant interferon trial in gastric cancer

1. Over-all survival and disease-free interval
2. Rate of local recurrences and distant metastases
3. Effects on immunological parameter (NIC-cells, T-ly-colonies) and natural hematopoiesis (CFU-C)
4. Relationship between cytotoxicity of IFN on gastric-cancer stem cells and the course of the disease

9th postoperative day with a dosis of 4×10^6 U twice a week for 4 months. The aim of this planned study is to elucidate what influence a postoperative adjuvant interferon therapy has on prolonging the relapse-free period or the survival time of gastric-cancer patients operated for potential cure. At the same time, a broad program of additional examinations was designed to investigate the influence of interferon on immunological in vitro parameters and hemopoesis (table II). In addition to this, an attempt is made to investigate a possible direct antiproliferative effect of interferon on the clonal tumor cell growth of gastric-cancer cells in vitro in individual patients, and to correlate this with the further course of the disease. Further statements about effects and side effects of interferon in the treatment of malignant tumors are expected from this program.

References

1 Editorial: What not to say about interferon. Nature *285:*603 (1980).
2 Gresser, J.; Tovey, M. G.: Antitumor effects of interferon. Bioch. biophys. Acta *516:*231 (1978).
3 Herfarth, Schlag (eds.), Gastric Cancer (Springer-Verlag, Berlin, Heidelberg, New York 1979).
4 Schlag, P.; Schreml, W.; Herfarth, C.: Antitumor activity of fibroblast interferon against human tumor cells in vitro (in print, 1981).

Prof. Ch. D. Herfarth, Department für Chirurgie, Universität Ulm, Steinhövelstr. 9, D-7900 Ulm-Safranberg

Interferon Therapy for Tumor Diseases in Man: Prospects for the Near Future

Hans Strander

Radiumhemmet, Karolinska Hospital, Stockholm, Sweden

Indroduction

Interferons (IFNs) constitute a family of proteins of which all are capable of exerting an antiviral action [1]. The proteins differ in their molecular composition; so far between 10 and 15 have been more or less well defined. They are able to act on single cells and on organs in both animals and man. They are involved in the regulatory systems of the body and have been applied in various important therapeutic contexts, among which the most familiar is the treatment of viral diseases and tumors [1 – 4].

Although IFNs can now be obtained in larger quantities than ever before, the world's total output this year is not likely to be sufficient for all clinical studies and prospective randomized trials designed to ascertain their effectiveness as antitumor agents. This paper outlines a number of points that merit consideration in clinical studies in the near future.

Types of Preparations

The main types of IFN that we are considering for clinical trials this year are listed in table I. Lymphoblastoid IFN are known to be heterogeneous. Various types of leukocyte IFN can be produced by *Escherichia coli*. There are possibly more than one kind of fibroblast IFN and there might be several types of immune IFN. The question

Table I. Main types of human IFN to be considered for clinical trials

Leu-α, leukocyte IFN
Ly-α, lymphoblastoid IFN
Coli-α, *E. coli* IFN of leukocyte type
Fib-β, fibroblast IFN
Coli-β, *E. coli* IFN of fibroblast type
Imm-γ, immune (type II) IFN
Coli-γ, *E. coli* IFN of immune type

whether the structural genes for human immune IFN can be inserted into *Escherichia coli* is at present being examined experimentally.

The number of IFNs present in all these preparations is very tentatively put at about 20. By recombination technology, hybrid molecules consisting of two IFNs have been produced. Thus, for our clinical trials we have to consider a large number of preparations. One must bear in mind, moreover, that, so far, all clinical work has been undertaken with impure preparations. The contaminants elicit immune responses, and this may lead to the induction of, for example, immune IFN, which might potentiate the action of the injected exogenous IFN.

The list may be extended to include the IFNs induced by injecting the stabilized polyIC-polyLysine.

Altogether some 10 IFNs will probably be tested in the near future for their antitumor effect in man. The number, in a few years, might well be doubled.

Internal Combinations

Various preparations of IFN may be combined. For instance, the inducers of IFN might be combined with exogenous IFN therapy, IFN-α could be combined with the β- or γ-types, and IFN-β with γ. In fact, all three of these types might be given to a particular patient. Various IFNs produced in *Escherichia coli* could be injected simultaneously, as could hybrid IFNs from *Escherichia coli*. Thus, the number of combinations of IFNs within the family that might be suitable for antitumor therapy in man is practically infinite. The main combinations are listed in table II.

Table II. Combinations of various types of IFN for clinical use

Inducers + IFN
$\alpha + \beta$
$\alpha + \gamma$
$\beta + \gamma$
$\alpha + \beta + \gamma$
Coli α-$_1$ + Coli α-$_2$
Coli hybrid combinations

Table III. Therapeutic variables

Disease
Disease stage
Purity of IFN
Dose
Routes of administration
Schedule
Comparisons to standard forms of treatment
Comparisons to IFN-α or -β
Duration of treatment
Order of treatments

External Combinations

The administration of any of the IFNs or inducers of IFN may also be combined with forms of treatment already given to tumor patients, the most common ones being chemotherapy, radiotherapy, and immunotherapy. Others include hormone therapy and hyperthermia. It must be emphasized that the choice of any particular standard treatment will depend on the type of tumor that the patient is suffering from. This would again lead to an endless number of combinations.

Therapeutic Variables

For any particular type of IFN used in a combination, either with others of the family or with other types of antitumor treatment, there is a large number of factors that may be varied. The most important of them are listed in table III. There are many benign and malignant *diseases* where therapy with IFN might be tried because the existing forms of treatment have proved to be of little benefit to the patient.

Therapy with IFN might be chosen for a particular *stage* of a disease – for example, at the microscopic or gross stage. The *purity* of the various preparations of IFN employed can be varied. There seems to have been no investigations of the possible importance of this factor. The *dose* of various types of IFN is another variable. We already have examples of tumor diseases where a low dose is ineffective but a higher one would probably prove beneficial. We also know that the type and degree of any side effects may depend on the dose.

The *route of administration* may be chosen according to the type of IFN being used. A classical example is the difference between the IFN-α- and β, which are given today by i.m. and i.v. injections, respectively. Which route is the most effective for any particular disease remains to be established.

The dose *schedule* may also be varied. In our osteosarcoma study, we give daily injections for the first month and then 3 times a week. However, this schedule, which was introduced as early as 1971, has no experimental basis.

In order to determine the efficacy of therapy with IFN under any particular set of conditions, the obtained results would have to be *compared* to those yielded by standard forms of treatment. This would require large-scale clinical trials which would take years to complete.

Comparisons must be made to ascertain whether the α-, β- and γ-types of IFN and the ones produced by *Escherichia coli* are better or worse than the types already being given to patients at this hospital.

Practically nothing is known about the required *duration of the therapy with IFN* in order to obtain benefit for a particular disease. In our studies on myeloma, we treat patients until complete remission has been achieved; and then for a further year. Some of our tumor patients have received IFN for 3 months, during which the disease progressed steadily. After a further 6 months of the same treatment, a regression was recorded. This emphasizes the importance of not ending IFN treatments after a short period. On the other hand, we do not know anything about the possible long-term side effects of several years of therapy with IFN.

The *order* in which IFN and other forms of treatments are given is another factor to be considered. The order of treatment might be extremely important; for example, it is not known whether patients given chemotherapy are likely to derive the full benefit of IFN. Nor do we know whether patients on IFN might later respond better or less well to chemotherapy than patients who have not received treatment previously. Nor do we know anything about the possible potentiating effects by combining various forms of treatment simultaneously.

Monitoring

The investigation of all these variables will entail an enormous amount of work at the clinical level. A central problem is that, at present, we are completely in the dark as to the principle mode of action of any of the IFNs in cases where regression of a tumor has been obtained. We know that various types of IFN can affect many body systems and possibly exert direct effects on tumor cells but we have no idea which effects are the most important ones. Without this knowledge it would be impossible to test patients before their treatment is begun. This is a classical problem common to all forms of tumor therapy. In the case of many diseases, we know from statistics and from experience for which patient a particular treatment is likely to be the most suitable one. Various methods for monitoring chemotherapeutic measures have recently been designed, but their development is at a preliminary stage.

The *side effects* observed after a patient has been given IFN may be examined, but we do not know whether they are due to IFN or to contaminants in the preparations. Again, the *level of IFN* in the patient's serum can be examined, but we do not know whether this variable has any bearing on the drug's therapeutic effect. Various types of *tumor cultures* can be designed, but for most tumors this is no easy matter. Short-term experiments on isotope incorporation can be performed to study the direct effects of the preparations on the patient's own tumor cells, and long-term cell cultures can be carried out, for example, by the agar colony technique in order to find whether or not the tumor is sensitive to IFN. Such studies would imply that the essential action of IFN in the tumor patient derives from a direct action on the tumor cells. Whether this is the case is not known.

Various *immunological variables* can also be examined; any of these undergo changes in the course of interferon therapy. Again, however, we do not know which of the immune factors, if any, have a bearing on the antitumor efficacy of a particular type of IFN.

Table IV. Monitoring of IFN effects

Side effects
Serum level of IFN
Short-term cell cultures
Long-term cell cultures
Immunological parameters
Antiviral assays
Production of IFN

Antiviral assays on patients receiving treatment with IFN is another possible approach. We have found, for example, that patients developing metastases despite treatment for microscopic osteosarcoma may contract subclinical and clinical viral infections during treatment with IFN. The reason for this is obscure, and the examination of a greater number of patients is required in order to see whether this variable merits study in clinical trials with IFN. Such a study would, however, have to be continued over a long period, by the end of which there might already be clinical evidence of the ineffectiveness of IFN therapy in such patients.

Screening for the *production of IFN* might be performed by artificial induction of IFN in cells taken from patients being treated with IFN or inducers of IFN. Whether there is any relationship between the induction level and the clinical effect is not known. Suggestions for monitoring are listed in table IV.

Prospects for the Future

This article outlines the complexity of, and some of the problems presented by clinical research aimed at designing the most effective type of IFN therapy for tumor patients. There is clearly a need for a deeper understanding of the mechanism underlying the action of interferon in tumor regression. Until this information is available, we shall still be fumbling in the dark and, for many of our patients, the therapy with IFN is likely to fall far short of the best conventional methods.

There is so far no conclusive evidence that therapy with IFN is better than conventional forms of treatment for the patient with a malignant tumor. This is hardly surprising in view of how little we know of the most favorable conditions for administering the drug.

Nonetheless, however remote the goal may seem to be at the present time, we have no alternative but to aim at it, if only because IFN may well offer a new and ultimately rewarding approach to the treatment of tumors in man.

References

1 Stewart, W. E.: The interferon system (Springer-Verlag, Wien-New York 1979).
2 Strander, H.: Interferons – Anti-neoplastic drugs? Blut *35:* 277–288 (1977).
3 Priestman, T. J.: Interferon: An anti-cancer agent? Cancer Treatm. Rev. *9:* 223–237 (1979).
4 Cantell, K.: Why is interferon not in clinical use today? Interferon *1:* 1–28 (1979).

Prof. Dr. Hans Strander, Karolinska Hospital, Radiumhemmet, S-10401 Stockholm 60